POTS Is Ruining My Life.

CW01431821

The Ultimate Guide to Finding Freedom From the Symptoms of Postural Orthostatic Tachycardia Syndrome

Leslie A. Harrington

To my mom, Laurice. My guardian angel, my person, and my believer who never left my side even when I didn't look sick. Thank you for teaching me to live by your daily words: "Do me proud." And to my dad, William, for teaching me a work ethic and encouraging my love for education and writing.

0

CHAPTER 1

PLEASE PASS THE SALT

"Never deny a diagnosis, but do deny the negative
verdict that may go with it."

– Norman Cousins

Several years ago, I was sitting at a health conference in Los Angeles, California watching a speaker engage the audience by challenging us to describe what we do in eight words or less. I thought, "That's impossible. What I do is way more complex than anything I could put into eight words!"

While I could have simply stated, "I am a transformational health coach," it doesn't truly capture what I do. A transformational health coach expands beyond simple nutrition and exercise. Transformation also encapsulates the mindset, psychology, connection, and spirituality. It is very personalized and incorporates the challenges of what motivates people for behavior change and how their thoughts about their health may be impacting their ability to enhance it. Rarely is one's capability to gain health ever simply about one thing.

I thought about when I was struggling with the diagnosis of POTS that left me with no answers and fending for myself. I thought about what I needed most back then when I had no support in the way of the medical world. I needed hope and answers. I needed to know my existence had not become about struggling to get through each day or wallowing in how sick I was feeling more often than not. I needed doctors who wanted to help fix me, not just patch my symptoms. I needed my health back and I needed the tools and guidance to restore it. I recalled the years I spent experimenting with what worked and what did not seem to have any impact at all.

Then I thought about each client that I work within my transformational health coaching practice – the work that we do together. I often call myself a "diagnosis strategist" because the client and myself are regularly working around a diagnosis, mostly POTS, and

2

the diagnosis is understandably the center of their existence. To move forward from the place of fear and into a place of action, we have to remove the elephant that is blocking the view of the road ahead. POTS defined every aspect of my life for years. There is no reason for others to waste ten years before they can live with a high quality of life in spite of a POTS diagnosis.

Each day, I witness and relate to clients describing their conditions and symptoms as part of how they identify themselves. They live by the words of doctors and have established their medication regimen to be permanent. They believe this is their life. They have adapted to feeling crummy most of the time. They have been led to believe there is very little they can do about POTS. They can only manage the symptoms and that is if they feel good enough to do just that.

They are enmeshed in their diagnosis. It runs every part of their activities. They slave to it each day to get the slightest relief. They are so focused on this diagnosis that their lives revolve around it. I know how this feels because, at one time, this was exactly how I would have described myself.

I support them in helping them realize, through the implementation of various lifestyle practices, there is more to life. We develop what that looks like together and we set out to reverse engineer the steps they can take to get there.

It is a decision and then a belief. A decision to separate from this second skin that holds the person back from believing in a better future. They have to remove the hat they wear with that diagnosis so boldly written across the top of their heads. I imagine taking off that hat and gently setting it down next to them so they can see it objectively. Or like wearing a prison jumpsuit and finally stepping out of it and letting it fall to the ground.

The process of healing had captured these images and results I had seen in myself and that I was seeing in my clients consistently. After all, this is the exact process I had to experience on my journey, and now I had the tools to help others to crawl out from under the very heavy label of POTS.

When I left the pharmacy industry, I jokingly told people, "I spent most of my career selling drugs, and I will spend the rest of my life helping get people off of them." I call this my Jekyll and Hyde personality: I

4

gained an understanding of one side of healthcare and then applied it to the other.

You don't need to be a scholar or change your career to take control of POTS symptoms, and you don't need to be an eternal optimist to find some good in a dark time. But what you can learn from others just like you is that the possibility to feel better is there, even if you have multiple diagnoses, pain, or disability. None of these people recognized what they were doing when they were doing it. They only knew how their relationship to POTS had changed, but technically, they very much had separated themselves from the limitations implied by their labels. You can too.

But before exploring *how*, let's talk a bit about what diagnosis is and isn't.

What is a diagnosis, anyway? Our lives are filled with labels. From the time we are children, we are identifying ourselves through the eyes of other people, most often our parents, from whom we desperately seek approval and significance. We label ourselves within the stories we create about ourselves. I was a smart kid. I was geeky with red hair, freckles, and Coke-bottle glasses. It's an identity I wore for years. Some people are labeled *popular* or *creative* or *artsy* or *athletic*. Labels can be good or bad and are just part of society's way of classifying people.

Diagnostic categories are similar. They're labels too; concepts, to put simply. Disease and syndrome labels are the same. A diagnosis attempts to determine which disease or condition explains a person's symptoms. Diagnostic labels are used to classify a person for research and treatment. The description helps professionals understand impairments and to discuss it with colleagues. Medical diagnoses are general labels that are constructed to convey a comprehension of illness. Diagnosis is just a tag, not a condemnation, nor does it cover the complexities of the human body. However, the idea of a label, especially created by a person in power, or a doctor, can create both external and internal stigma.

In theory, the diagnosis should direct your course of treatment. It would potentially provide a framework that would include the medications you take, your treatment protocol, and possible prognosis. Note that a diagnosis does not mean *defective*. If we look at it as a road map to identifying a plan and we reverse engineer the origin of the first symptom, we may be able to navigate to the destiny of restored health more effectively.

Unfortunately, although a diagnosis is a starting point from a medical point of view, it's used frequently as a shorthand and sometimes a shortcut – a way to describe a person. And that's when it carries the danger of becoming a permanent label, both to the individual living with the label and to the community surrounding them.

For example, let's look at insurance. Your insurance coverage is determined by your diagnosis "code." Typically, insurance covers only what is medically necessary. Without a diagnostic code, you may be rejected for a claim. Doctors want you to get the treatment that won't bankrupt you, so what do they do? They may look at a complex list of symptoms and pick a code that allows you to take the next step. The politics of insurance might land you a diagnosis that is convenient for payment (and send you on a stressful or even wrong path in the process).

I often hear the following joking comment, which rings with so much truth: "If you can name it, you can blame it." Once you receive a name for a condition, you can now place the responsibility on the diagnosis for hosting all of your health challenges. Similarly, this expression hints at drugs being the solution for symptom control. As the public, we are consumers of medications, but often we aren't aware of how the diagnosis, coding, and labels can work in favor of or against getting financial support from your insurance policy.

One of the problems with a diagnosis is that people often assume an all-or-nothing approach: I have it or I don't. However, not every diagnosis is life-long. Even if yours is considered "incurable" or not likely to be changed or corrected, it certainly does not mean you are now defined by this new label. You did not go from *you* one day to a different version of *you* the next day simply because of the assignment of a diagnosis. This all-or-nothing thinking gets in the way of so many aspects of life because it leaves no room for compromise. It's the sense of *I am this or I am that* versus the ability to live in a place of more than one truth that limits the expression of your whole personality. If you can't view life from various perspectives, you are stuck in tunnel vision. Black-and-white thinking forces you to live in

8

extremes, but illness often doesn't work that way. One of the benefits of understanding POTS is that you'll open up your thinking to include the shades of gray, so you add tools to help keep you in balance.

POTS, therefore, is a simple bucket. It conceivably serves more purpose for physicians and insurance companies than it does for a patient. A diagnosis is not a conclusion. A diagnosis is not an imperfection. It doesn't have to be a shortcoming. And, most definitely, it is not a fate. A diagnosis is a component of the exquisite journey of life.

WHAT THE HECK IS POTS?

POTS is an acronym for Postural Orthostatic Tachycardia Syndrome. The term POTS was established in 1993, but the illness has been known throughout history by other names. In the past, it was thought to be caused by anxiety, but more recently, it has become clear this is not the case. POTS is a malfunction of the autonomic nervous system (ANS). The causes of this malfunction can be any number of things. POTS is not considered a disease; rather, it is a syndrome or *a cluster of symptoms frequently seen together*.

According to Dysautonomia International, POTS is a form of dysautonomia (dysfunction of the ANS) that is estimated to affect between 1 million and 3 million Americans. There are millions of more cases around the world. POTS is most commonly seen in women (approximately eighty percent of cases) between the ages of fifteen and fifty.

POTS is very personal and can affect people very differently. Therefore, the cause, type of POTS, treatment, and prognosis should also be personal. The treatment of POTS has become more standard. The recommendation includes a dramatic increase of fluid intake and over triple the daily consumption of salt, compression socks, other means to improve blood flow, and avoidance of situations or exposure to the threat of things that could worsen symptoms. For me, that could be hot temperatures, various foods, barometric pressure, air travel, or lack of exercise/movement. Stress proved to be a huge promoter of symptoms. I wish I had realized this earlier. Various prescription medications are used to treat each symptom.

10

The problem with the common treatment is that one size does not fit all. The medications cause other harmful effects on the body that can ultimately exaggerate the symptoms of POTS. The sodium intake should be considered from a clean source. There are often nutrient deficiencies associated with POTS, and the conventional world does not often suggest supplementation. Understanding how to find the right type of supplement and know that it is safe to take is extremely important. Things like adaptogenic herbs, magnesium, and chlorophyll are never mentioned in any of the material you read on POTS. These little gems were life-changing for me and essential to aiding me to get off of my many supposed *life-long* medications. I'll talk about this in more detail in the lifestyle and nutrition chapter.

One feature of POTS that is universally present is *cardiovascular deconditioning*. Another characterization involves hypovolemia, a decreased volume of blood in the body or a loss of extracellular fluid. The symptoms of hypovolemia coincide with POTS symptoms such as headache, fatigue, weakness, dizziness, or thirst.

DIAGNOSTIC CRITERIA OF POTS

The diagnostic criteria of POTS primarily focus on the increase in heart rate upon standing, but the complexity of other symptoms is the biggest challenge. Besides hypovolemia, POTS patients tend to have higher levels of norepinephrine when standing which signifies the presence of increased sympathetic nervous system activation. Essentially, a person with POTS is more often in the "fight or flight" mode of the nervous system than is normal or necessary. Therefore, it leads to a prolonged or sensitive stress response. Other common symptoms include lightheadedness, heart palpitations, exercise intolerance, heat intolerance, chest pain, decreased concentration (brain fog), nausea, tremors, syncope (fainting), coldness in the extremities, chest pain, and shortness of breath. Still another fifty percent of POTS patients experience an impact on their sudomotor nerves which is associated with sweating.

The range of debilitation between those diagnosed with POTS is wide. In some, the quality of life may be compared to that of a person with COPD or

12

congestive heart failure. Sadly, it is also compared to that of a person on dialysis for kidney failure. On the flip side, there is over seventy-five percent of POTS patients who can function on some working level. Many can work and have a somewhat normal social life. Others may have significant disruption to activities in daily life that involve the upright position for extended periods. Some see fluctuation or experience *flare-ups*.

The exciting news is that researchers believe that some POTS patients will continue to see improvement over time. There is not a lot of long term studies related to the course of POTS, but that is why I am writing this book. I am a long-term study. There is hope. The prognosis is good for most patients, especially if you can identify an underlying cause. That is where I never gave up the search and where functional medicine plays a crucial role. You will learn more about functional medicine in future chapters.

SUBTYPES AND ASSOCIATED CONDITIONS OF POTS:

1. POTS characterized by high flow, low flow, and normal flow (blood) standing decent of blood. High is a significant flow movement from the thoracic cage (rib area) to the lower extremities.

2. Neuropathies: a loss of function in lower extremities. More than fifty percent of POTS patients express these symptoms. Characterized by peripheral sympathetic denervation impaired vasoconstriction, increase venous pooling (blood pools in the legs), which makes it difficult for the blood to return to the heart from the legs.

3. Hyperadrenergic POTS: approximately thirty percent of POTS patients. Elevated standing norepinephrine, which is the driver of excessive tachycardia palpitations, hyperhidrosis, abdominal pain, and nausea. The symptoms are exaggerated with physical exertion and emotional stress.

4. Mast cell activation disorder (MCAD): the inappropriate release of histamine and other mast cell activators in response to physical activity or orthostatic stress. Elevated plasma tryptase during a POTS episode or high level of

14

histamines. The symptoms include flushing, shortness of breath, headaches, light headiness, digestive distress, and excessive diuresis (urination).

When looking for a root cause of POTS, it is really important to understand the various other conditions that may be one way or another related to POTS:

1. Autoimmunity: in some patients, POTS appears following vital illness or family history of autoimmunity.

2. Volume of blood circulation: thirty percent exhibit clinical evidence of hypovolemia.

3. Effect of sex and the menstrual cycle: there is evidence of fluctuations in symptoms during a women's cycle when estrogen and progesterone are dropping. This change is presumably related to the balance of testosterone and estrogen.

4. Diurnal variability: a variation in the output of a substance. POTS patients tend to have worse symptoms in the morning, likely because they have gone a long period lying down with no fluids.

5. Bed rest and deconditioning: many studies demonstrated deconditioning even in healthy individuals. This may be why the positive response to exercise is so striking.

OTHER DIFFERENTIAL DIAGNOSIS AND ASSOCIATED CONDITIONS:

1. Vasovagal syncope: a condition that leads to fainting in some people, often caused by the body's overreaction to certain triggers.
2. Neurogenic orthostatic hypotension (NOH): sometimes seen in people with Parkinson's, multiple systems atrophy, and other neuropathies.
3. Inappropriate sinus tachycardia: The heart-racing occurs independently of body position, such as nighttime supine (lying down, face up) tachycardia.
4. Pheochromocytoma: adrenal gland tumor located on top of the kidneys. Symptoms are not positional and plasma mechanisms not elevated when dealing with this condition.
5. Chest sinus tachycardia: typical of anemia, anxiety, infection, or fever. Activation of the sympathetic

nervous system and the deactivation of the parasympathetic.

6. Any type of structural cardiac disease. Hypotension (low blood pressure) or tachycardia alone.

MORE IMPORTANT SYMPTOMS AND CONDITIONS TO CONSIDER FOR DIFFERENTIAL DIAGNOSIS FOR POTS

1. Migraines, G.I. disorders, fibromyalgia, chronic fatigue, etcetera may or may not be associated

2. Ehlers-Danlos syndrome and hyper-mobility frequently occur with POTS. Be open to the possibility of impairment of connective tissue, which may lead to abnormalities in vascular compliance and increase leg blood pooling.

3. Migraine and brain trauma or contusion. Increased sympathetic activity may contribute to frequencies of headaches, however, the head injuries can lead to bed rest.

4. Hypervigilance and anxiety. Symptomatology increases dramatically without any other reason.

17

5. Chronic fatigue and fibromyalgia, very frequent in POTS. About fifty percent of POTS patients have chronic fatigue. Such patients with chronic fatigue and fibromyalgia tend to have small hearts and excessive sympathetic activation which often results in a reduction of physical activity. This domino effect leads to subsequent deconditioning and exaggeration of orthostatic intolerance.

6. Brain fog is a cognitive complaint similar to that of mental fatigue. It presents worse with poor sleep.

7. Increase daytime sleepiness and sleep disturbance.

8. GI dysmotility: bloating, nausea, vomiting, abdominal pain, constipation, and diarrhea are all common in POTS because autonomic imbalance leads to abnormal gastric emptying.

9. Chronic pelvic pain and overactive bladder. Increased daytime frequency and urgency which may be related to drinking more water.

POTS is a paradox. A diagnosis of POTS simple, but to manage it is very complex.

HOW IS POTS DIAGNOSED?

Currently, POTS is diagnosed using the criteria of a heart rate increase of thirty beats per minute (bpm) or more (or over 120 bpm) within the first ten minutes of standing, in the absence of orthostatic hypotension. This means without a drop in blood pressure at the same time as the increase in heart rate.

A tilt table test is also a standard measurement for POTS. Alternatively, you may simply have your blood pressure and heart rate measured in the laying-down and standing-up positions at two-minute, five-minute, and ten-minute intervals.

Other tests that measure ANS function are also considered. Tests such as the quantitative sudomotor axon reflex test (QSART), thermoregulatory sweat test (TST), and even skin biopsies to test tissue.

All of the information I have reported above can be found at https://dysautonomiainternational.org [1] and the American College of Cardiology, JACC Podcast [2].

That is about as formal as I will get when it comes to all things POTS. The rest comes from experience, taking chances, personal failures and wins, experimentation, research, studying, doctors, hospitals, specialists and lots and lots of time. I talk about many tools that I could have never imagined would help so substantially with the POTS symptoms. Some I picked up through recommendations, therapeutic settings, or my elimination process. Reminding yourself that you don't have to have it all one way or another is helpful on this journey.

It is easy to get sucked into POTS to the extent it becomes all-consuming. Holding your constant attention to what's wrong in your body steals from the joy of other aspects of life. While self-care is imminent when you must put all of your effort into your health, losing sight of other aspects of life may harm your efforts of returning to stability.

When we think of the word "balance," we imagine equal parts or symmetry. In the attempt to find balance in health, work, home, social life, and personal growth, we wind up with the pressure of needing to be in sync in all areas at all times. This is just not realistic. In life, there will be times when work will require more from you. Other times, your family will be the only thing that matters. When your health is off, the focus may need to shift to change your priorities. The word "harmony" feels more flowing. To adapt and adjust, gracefully transitioning from one area to another as needed, may be more ideal than trying to perfect balance.

For example, when I was first diagnosed with POTS, I was overly-involved in my diagnosis, which was where I needed to be to get well. That is until my mom was diagnosed with cancer and my focus shifted to supporting her. Suddenly, my stability just had to happen with less of an intense focus for me to be there in her time of need. And it did. My tools were effective even when I wasn't staring at them constantly. They had become a non-negotiable part of my day and life, and I didn't notice that they still happened in spite of my attention to other things.

Because of the tools, I was able to shift more of my energy outside of myself to honor my mom. I am still amazed by how the universe had my back. Work, which was always crazy, suddenly slowed and began to run smoothly, freeing me up to go to Mom's chemo sessions and drive her to doctor's appointments. When she finished chemo, things picked back up and I got back to being busy in the office. When things took that next turn for the worse, work took a back seat. Incredibly, as I allowed things to flow as they had to (and I had no choice except to ride the waves), it lessened the resistance and allowed that harmony that can even be found in the most difficult of times. I still snuck in trips to the ER for fluids and I relied on my meds back then, but I was forced to see that when something else became more blaring, POTS took the back seat. It had to.

FINDING A HIGH QUALITY OF LIFE IN SPITE OF POTS

I love how motivational speaker Lisa Nichols explains the world of duality in which we live. She says that there are always two parts to everything in life, and people tend to forget we have the opportunity to live in the space of both. This is a blessing!

For example, you get to be brilliant at that which you are great at. You also get to be an amateur and not know what you don't know. But this lack of knowledge does not take away from or threaten your brilliance. As Lisa says, "You get to be amazing, and you get to be confused. You get to be awesome and have those moments of ADD. You get to be strong, but you get to be held. You get to be courageous, but you get to be fearful. As long as you allow yourself to live in the duality, we get to have all of you."

Embracing duality is permitting yourself to have moments that feel defeating and then moments in which nothing can stop you. You'll have moments in which you are convinced "you got this" and moments when you may need someone to remind you of your strength.

Healing through POTS encompasses duality. To know strength is to have felt weakness. To know courage is to have fallen in fear. To know separation, you must have once been entangled. Just because you strive to become independent of the label does not mean the symptoms cease to exist altogether. It means you get to be powerful in conjunction with embracing vulnerability.

I began to see that each person I worked with in practice was struggling with the exact challenges of someone who was diagnosed with POTS, someone who had reached the end of their rope, someone who was losing hope and only knew this new way of living. I

23

maintain that following the steps and making promises to yourself that you will commit to consistently implement these tools will take you down the road to healing, regardless of your diagnosis code.

To progress, you must be able to see yourself feeling well. You must *believe* in the prospect of enjoying life again. We tend to get stuck in the belief that this is it, this is our new reality. That mentality has to shift. POTS is not your destiny!

When someone is sick, they have one goal – to regain health or to feel better. When someone has their health, they have many goals. I often begin a session working with clients by asking two questions:

- When was the last time you recall feeling amazing?

- If I could wave a magic wand and grant you a perfect day where you feel healthy and amazing, what would that look like for you? How would you feel? How would you spend your time?

It would make me so sad to hear most of them answer both questions by saying, "I have no idea." It had been so long since they felt well, not only can they not remember when it was, they cannot imagine what it will feel like to ever feel good again.

On the other hand, they may know exactly the time and place in which they felt good, but it was fifteen years ago. It was a very specific time or event that surrounded the turning point in their health. It is even more engrained there is no hope because they are so used to feeling like crap.

I am always shocked by how many people don't know what it would look like or feel like to have a great day. Worse, if they recall when they felt amazing last, it's almost always very distinct and in the very distant past. As they began to fill their toolbox, each person was able to implement them into their journey in various ways until they felt that transitional time when things began to shift.

The more tools you have, the duration in which you may suffer declines, the time between those painful spots begins to get longer, and the frequency of episodes is fewer.

As Tony Robbins says, "Where focus goes, energy flows." It's easy to underestimate the power of focus. After all, most of the time we are running on autopilot. Our thoughts shift to places and before we know it, we believe our nonsense. We can drown in the negativity if we don't tap into the awareness of our thoughts.

When I became aware, I started to hear myself complain. I expected what was going to come next. I assumed – because one day in one moment, I had a response to a particular trigger, whether it was food, lack of sleep, a shower that was too hot, one less glass of water – that I would experience that same symptom again. Often, I did. It's more likely because I was seeking out validation for my beliefs. If I knew I was going to feel crappy, my brain happily granted me the satisfaction of proving me right.

Of course, my body's responses came about unexpectedly, especially in the beginning. But now, if something taps me on the shoulder, I know better. I am confident it's going to be all good because I can work through it both physically and mentally.

I have a choice. I can focus on all of my symptoms or I can focus on how it will feel to get back in harmony with my body.

It is not going to be positive all of the time. But the more aware we are of our negative self-chatter, the quicker you can thought-shift and redirect your focus.

When those moments of disappointment, sadness, or setbacks happen, know that it's temporary. Life happens in waves. It will never be all great or all bad. But it will always be an opportunity for growth and learning. Be grateful for the lessons. Often, the things that we love come out of our suffering.

My best friend has these little one-liners that have stuck with me throughout my life. "The best predictor of future behavior is past behavior," she says. This one seems obvious, but to many, it is not that clear. Think about it. Behavior change is hard. I mean really hard. Many people live their lives getting more of the same.

When faced with situations that require significant changes to one's core habit loop, patterns of daily life, or a shift in mindset, this is no easy accomplishment. The way we behave through life is somewhat static, generally speaking. As Brené Brown tells us, "Vulnerability sounds like truth and feels like courage. Truth and courage aren't always comfortable, but they're never weakness." We will discuss practices

27

to help better create behavior change in the upcoming chapters.

YOU ARE NOT YOUR DIAGNOSIS

I remember exactly where I was and what I was feeling during a routine run with my dog, when I randomly stumbled on a podcast I did not typically listen to. I'll never forget this one phrase that was very powerful and became one of my mantras: "You are not your pain." When I first went off my medication for arthritis in my knees, I repeated this phrase in my head. You're not defined by any situation. I knew my pain wasn't who I was. It wasn't connected to me personally. I would tell myself that two weeks ago when I was on the medication, my knees were the same as they are today.

"You are not your pain" came to be a force in my mindset. Pain is not a choice, but suffering is. Thinking about the thing that haunts you the most and constantly focusing on it only draws you closer to it. Eventually, my mind wrapped around the concept of my pain not being my pain. It was pain, but it did not belong to me. It was real pain but it was different now because of the way I viewed it.

When people describe their situation as "my arthritis," "my Crohn's," or "my diabetes," they are owning it like it defines who they are or as if it gives them a title.

I would say to myself repeatedly, "This isn't me. This isn't who I am."

I am not my POTS!

The goal of this book is to help you to be in control of the symptoms of POTS. This new-found freedom opens so many doors to expand your quality of life and pursue your life goals in spite of living with POTS.

It took me years to free my body and my mind from POTS, and I am here to help you find a more direct path to healing. I've taken all the medications. I did all of the things the conventional doctors recommended. It was not enough. I was just simply going through the robotic motions of life. Until I created my standard of care and ongoing maintenance that has proven itself effective time and again. I'll begin by telling you a little about my story and how I came to learn the shortcuts and facts about dealing with a POTS diagnosis.

CHAPTER 2

THE POTS PUZZLE

"Do the best you can until you know better. Then, when you know better, do better."

– Maya Angelou

LIFE BEFORE AND AFTER POTS

Have you ever known something was physically wrong with your health but no doctor or professional could tell you exactly what was happening? You may have gone through a dramatic, ongoing investigation involving tests and rule-outs and still come up empty-handed.

On that day when the one doctor finally put a name to your so-called "ailment," you suddenly felt

31

relieved. But that name or label was just the beginning of your journey. Living under the new diagnosis may have quickly turned into *becoming* the diagnosis – and losing yourself. That's what happened to me.

In 2009, I was a thirty-five-year-old career girl living the life of a road warrior as a corporate sales director for a generic pharmaceutical distributor. I loved my job, even though the travel was taking its toll on me. It was a fast-paced, high-stress career in which everything was deemed an emergency. Getting away for the weekend was about the only vacation I ever saw in my work life. Therefore, when my roommate, Kelly, and I decided to go to Key West, I was thrilled.

We spent our first day soaking up the sun at our quaint little hotel pool followed by a dinner overlooking the coast of Florida. The worries of the world washed away as we inhaled the endless, salty ocean and watched the sunset with some other friends. Walking down Duval Street, we stopped into Sloppy Joe's Bar where the music was blaring and the place was overflowing with a mix of locals and even more tourists. Kelly left to use the bathroom while I waited for her at the bar. At that moment, I felt inclined to watch my drink. I put my hand over it as if to shield it from an invisible threat.

A sort of grungy, older guy was standing to the right side of me at the bar. He struck up a conversation beginning with, "You look bored." He must have noticed my disinterest because he soon pulled out his wallet and proceeded to show me pictures of his disabled child. She was a beautiful, young girl in a wheelchair. It was instinctual for me to ask questions and engage in dialogue. Kelly returned and we were both ready to head out. As we paid the tab, the man at the bar stopped me and said, "You don't look bored anymore."

I walked away thinking the comment was strange, but I shook it off. Before hopping in the cab, I threw out my half-full drink.

Half the drink was all it took. We were almost back to the hotel just a few short miles from the bar when I began laughing uncontrollably. No jokes, no prompting, nothing funny. By the time we arrived at the hotel, I knew something was very wrong.

I finally blacked out. I don't remember the rest of the night or the entire next morning. Kelly packed our bags and loaded the car while I laid uselessly. I only remember feeling like I was in a terrible fog but not a typical hangover fog. I had never felt this before.

My parents met me at my house to take me to the hospital. When we arrived and got checked in, the emergency-room doctor explained that the hospital did not test for street drugs, only cocaine and marijuana. She said if these drugs came up in my bloodwork, it would "look bad on the insurance." They added that anyway, there was nothing they could do for me since it had been over twelve hours since I had been exposed to the drug. The doctor advised that I would be better off taking an over-the-counter drug test from Walgreens next time. She sent us away citing "stomach pain" on my ER report.

My parents were shaken. I was a mess. I felt embarrassed and ashamed but still so grateful that I was with my friend and hadn't been physically harmed by the person who poisoned me.

The next day, I noticed when I turned my head, the room would slowly follow at its own pace like a trailing vision. I was still loopy and confused. My brain felt damaged. I feared I would never get my brain cells back. I immediately noticed feeling dizzy. My heart was pounding out of my chest. I felt exhausted more often than not.

After two weeks of these symptoms, I realized something in my body had broken. However, it would be six months after the incident in the Keys before my diagnosis was clear.

My general practitioner doctor reported I was likely out of shape. I thought to myself, "If this is what out of shape feels like, I will never be out of shape again." When a doctor tells you *nothing* is wrong, it can be just as powerful as when they tell you *something* is wrong. You find yourself doing "normal" things that feel dangerous. You know what you're doing doesn't feel right, but because someone told you it's okay, you do it.

My physician was right about one thing: I was not in good shape at the time. My best stress-relief was a bottle of wine. My nutrition choices were less than stellar. And I didn't remember the last time I stepped foot in a gym. I decided to hire a trainer and work out. Against every grain in my body, I also began walk/jogging, even though I felt with every step I was going to pass out. But the doctor said I was out of shape, so…I attempted to ignore the symptoms and pushed myself through.

The doctor had said I was fine. I wasn't fine. I struggled to get through every workout. I gasped through my runs, stopping frequently to slow down my heart. The south Florida heat was intolerable. I felt *off* every day of the week. The dizziness and heart-racing breathlessness were the most profound symptoms. I was always on the verge of blacking out. I was an avid equestrian in those days; riding horses was my passion. Suddenly, riding became hard for me. One day, I got overheated while riding. My heart rate soared to over 170 bpm. Over thirty minutes after my ride was over and I had just been sitting down cooling off, my heart was still pounding at 120 bpm. I started to panic, unsure why it wasn't coming down. In my frenzy, my heart raced even more, which landed me in the emergency room. The ER doctor took my vitals but he also tried something different. He took my blood pressure and pulse while I was lying down, sitting, and standing up. He confirmed my pulse rate shifted as I changed positions, and it didn't shift just a little, but by as many as thirty points!

He also saw an abnormality on my EKG and wanted me to see an electrophysiologist to be certain the abnormality wasn't causing my symptoms. An

36

electrophysiologist is a type of cardiologist that deals more with electrical aspects of the heart. They treat heart rhythm problems. Two months after the Key West drugging, I finally had someone take me seriously. Unfortunately, this would not be the norm. After that day, I never found another ER doctor or any other practitioner who took the time to understand my symptoms. I always looked fine on paper, but inside, I was in complete disarray. Still, what choice did I have but to follow the doctor's orders?

After that ER visit, I went to see the recommended electrophysiologist. He advised me to eat three tablespoons of salt per day. Yes, *tablespoons!* He explained that when I drink four bottles of water, my body believes I drank only one. "It is like running on a gas tank that is always half empty," he said. He didn't explain why or how this happened; only that it is what my body was doing. While the drugging incident was certainly correlated, he downplayed the involvement and focused on my symptoms rather than the cause. The electrophysiologist told me the headaches I experienced were a mild sign of dehydration. The salt and water he prescribed helped increase the volume of my blood so it

37

pumped more efficiently. Lots of salt equals increased blood pressure. If the salt wasn't effective enough, I experienced nausea and dizziness until it felt like the room would blackout, though not quite to the point of fainting. He prescribed me a heart medication to help with the tachycardia (the racing of my heart) as well as a medication for nausea.

Next, he scheduled me for the tilt table test. During the test, he and the nurse strapped me to a table and injected my veins with adrenaline. Then they electronically tilted the table to an upright position to see if I would faint. They measured my heart rate during and after the transition. The doctor informed me that this was the standard test for a condition called POTS. POTS is a dysfunction of the ANS, and it presents as a collection of symptoms.

Based on the results of this test and my other textbook symptoms, I finally had an answer, and POTS was its name! Why is there a sense of relief when we get someone to validate us with a diagnosis? It's like it gives the situation a legitimacy it lacked before the name.

When I was drugged, he said, the regular processes that occurred in my body day-to-day (pupils dilating, body temperature variations, heart rate changing, blood pressure rising and falling) no longer occurred automatically. These natural processes have a regulatory system that keeps them balanced: the autonomic nervous system. You never have to think about them happening; they just do. The same goes for your body's fight-or-flight mode, or when your body feels stress – some processes shut off, and others turn on, but you maintain regulation. My body stopped doing that for me.

This was what POTS meant: my body no longer maintained homeostasis.

I soon learned that with POTS, you need a team. This initial electrophysiologist was one of the three I had visited. I also saw several cardiologists, a neurologist, and even an allergist!

In my early days of POTS, I spent a lot of time in the hospital, especially during the first six months after the diagnosis. I didn't have a system in place right away. My toolbox was pretty empty initially, and I learned the hard way that my body needed the most. Because I wasn't sure how to describe my symptoms, a plethora of testing was ordered for me, but it was all repetitive of things I already knew were in the clear. Doctors always ordered heart testing initially because of the tachycardia and the slight EKG variance. It became annoying to go into clinics and have to wait for the doctors to do their due diligence, discovering what I already knew wasn't wrong.

Fortunately, down the road, after I had learned some of the skills to manage POTS, I met my soon-to-be favorite electrophysiologist, Dr. Kenisberg. He would be the physician who was most clear about how to manage POTS. I recited my habits and symptom-management techniques to him. I was surprised when he said, "That's all you can do." I was hoping he would give me some secret to help me get POTS out of my world. He commended me on my routine and my exercise and seemed sad that more people couldn't get to the place where I was currently functioning. By then, I was exercising regularly, eating a clean diet, ingesting my oodles of salt, hydrating, taking my medications (which was up to four at this point) and learning everything I could about POTS. I was also in my fifth year of suffering from the symptoms of POTS.

While he didn't offer me a resolution, he seemed unaffected by the lack of knowledge around the syndrome. He sent me home with the book *The Fainting Phenomenon: Understanding Why People Faint and What to Do about It*. This book contained more direction than I had been given through the entire process.

Think about that. Perhaps you've experienced something similar in your life. At first, the book was frustrating, but frustration quickly changed to gratitude in the process of reading it. I felt more educated than I had in my original research on POTS. This, in part, was because POTS was so new and misunderstood that there was not a lot written about it. The book explained the dynamics of the ANS, which allowed me to understand POTS differently.

I had been told I was out of shape and that I should eat salt and drink more water. Then I was given a book. Since it was a syndrome or collection of symptoms, there was no single treatment. Everywhere I turned, I was faced with the same feedback: POTS was my fate.

After that, I developed a personal POTS routine.

During a flare-up, there always came a point when I knew if I could work through the symptoms or if I wouldn't be able to recover on my own.

If I couldn't pull it together or knew I had travel or something else was coming up that would set me back, a trip to the ER was to get fluids. These days were easy to spot; even if I had a free-flowing fountain and drank water from morning to night, everything would begin to shut down. I would get nauseous. My symptoms of heart-racing and dizziness were exaggerated. I had trouble walking without feeling like I might pass out. None of my "tricks" worked. The salt and water did nothing. The medication was not effective. Even the anti-nausea pill wasn't helpful. Then my bladder would kick in: I would be full of salt and water but unable to urinate. My digestion would lock up. I couldn't break down food and I would have severe stomach pain. The entire "rest and digest" part of my nervous system would shut down.

These flare-ups happened at least one time each month in the first year of the diagnosis of POTS and would last for many days. In subsequent years, as I began to heal my body, I saw the frequency shift and the intensity lessen. But until that point, I was dealing with these fierce times routinely.

This was my life now. Frustrated and discouraged but determined at the same time, I set out to embrace this new lifestyle. I now faced my day with acceptance. I shook hands with my symptoms. In my new lifestyle, I simply accepted that POTS was part of me.

OWNING POTS

POTS was officially *mine*. *My* POTS dictated my days: my activities, my work life, my social life, and, of course, my private life. I didn't go anywhere without my POTS. Even if I woke up feeling fantastic and had a great workout, POTS was always a part of my conversations. I regularly spoke of POTS, defending it and explaining how it controlled every part of my body.

POTS did not like to be told what to do. I was a slave to POTS. I had not overcome it. I had not won any fights; I had simply learned to turn the other cheek. I adjusted my *response* to my symptoms. They had not subsided or taken a break. My condition was consistent in its ability to run the day.

My activities became more isolated, I grew more withdrawn, losing myself somewhere in my routine life. I forgot what fun was like. I didn't know the freedom of spontaneity anymore. If someone questioned my relationship, I defended it. *I fought for my limitations, instead of fighting to go beyond them.* I became POTS. It owned me.

When I began lying to myself and others, I realized my life was going in an unhealthy direction. For example, once I realized the keywords that made people stop questioning my choices, I ran with it. I claimed I was "allergic" to things I was afraid to eat. I warned that other things made me violently ill, which wasn't entirely untrue but was a dramatic description. I couldn't distinguish between the things that I truly couldn't tolerate anymore. I had trained my brain to fear anything that I deemed not good for me.

I reported that I felt too sick to go out on most nights, conveniently when it was something I just didn't feel like doing. I didn't feel like explaining myself. I blamed my condition for everything. It served me in such a negative way, detrimental to my potential of ever-rising above it and beating it.

One night, I went out with a friend. I came home and was brushing my teeth to prepare for bed when my last heart medication pill fell on the floor. I panicked. I fell to my knees, looking everywhere, thinking I would be doomed if I missed this dose. I was crying and frantically searching for the pill when suddenly I looked at myself in the mirror: I felt like an addict. I was convinced this pill was so powerful that a single missed dose would completely turn my life upside-down.

What was happening to me? Was I addicted to a non-addictive substance? I was addicted to the idea that this pill dictated how I felt for the day. I was addicted to what the doctors told me when I asked how long I had to take the medications: "For the rest of your life." That thought frightened me. I had been telling myself and others a story, one that I was writing as I went.

I changed in other ways too.

Exercise became my passion – an opportunistic word for obsession. If I didn't get out of bed and get my blood flowing first thing in the morning, my day would be in shambles. I would step out of bed and raise my

45

hands over my head to see if my blood was flowing. Then I would wait for the fog to come over me. It was the feeling of darkness you get when you stand up too fast. This was my test: how black my vision was would determine how I proceeded.

Because food was an issue (I'd developed a sugar and alcohol intolerance), I logged and carefully monitored my heart after eating different foods and doing various workouts and at numerous times of the month.

I even had my heart rate tested by a professional to see what my body's normal maximum rate was. The average maximum heart rate calculation is 220 minus your age. This is the maximum number of times your heart should beat per minute during exercise. My heart rate tested equivalent to that of a nine-year-old: 211 beats per minute, and that was *on* medication. My working zone heart rate was a zone most people couldn't hit without collapsing.

I used this knowledge to bump my fitness level up a notch. Understanding that 211 was normal for me and I didn't have to be afraid of being in the high 190s during a workout (because my doctors said it was okay!),

I was able to adapt to the scary feeling of the racing heart and push myself while assuming I was improving my fitness. I learned how to maximize my high-intensity workouts to give me the best blood flow and increase oxygen, so I could make it through my day. I never missed a workout.

Over time, I developed many theories around POTS. I became a symptom-management expert and was more mindful of my body.

Thirty pounds lighter and in *the best shape of my life*, I found myself in my mid-thirties on four prescription drugs. I was calculated, concise, and regimented – but I had become somewhat of a different person. All of this hard work lessened my hospital visits, although the symptoms still got the best of me at times.

As it turned out, my medications were part of what was keeping me sick.

After I was drugged in Key West, I struggled with receiving a lot of different advice from doctors. I was prescribed drugs as if they were patches to put on all the symptoms I was experiencing. The medications ranged from heart pills for the tachycardia, anti-nausea pills, a vasodilator that increased my blood pressure when it dropped too low, to vertigo medication for the dizziness. There truly is a "pill for every ill."

Wanting to know more about what I was taking, I reached out to my pharmacy partners, asking them to help me understand how these drugs should have been helping me recover. They were very supportive, but I noticed they wouldn't take these drugs if faced with the option themselves.

Nobody in my industry wanted to be on drugs of any kind. They were selling the drugs, prescribing them to patients, and creating and manufacturing them, but they wouldn't touch them with a ten-foot pole. I found that interesting and disturbing.

I was tired of the routine medication refill appointments and not seeing any real change in my prognosis. The next piece of news I received was alarming. My cardiologist had announced randomly in one of my check-ups that I needed to "watch my sugar." I seriously thought he had the wrong chart. I asked for a history of my blood sugar readings and it was clear: I was prediabetic. My blood sugar (A1C reading) had been creeping up from 5.7 to 5.8 to 5.9 over the past nine months, when I was at my lightest weight and did not eat

48

sugar or any starchy carbs, let alone anything processed or bad for me. How could this be?

THE TURNING POINT

During this daily routine of keeping my head above water and addressing my new *problem*, my family received terrible news. My dear mom, Laurice, was diagnosed with bladder cancer. The next several months would be filled with surgery, chemotherapy, transfusions, medical negligence, and downright horrific sickness. I felt so helpless. At the same time, my father was also ill with ongoing conditions including high blood pressure, congestive heart failure, and diabetes.

Being with them during their decline was a devastating time, to say the least. But witnessing my parents' illnesses provided distance from my story and a turning point in how I thought about my problems. My mother's fight with cancer in particular provided perspective.

One day during her illness, I was going for a run. I felt dizzy and light-headed, but there was always a point in my run when I became a bit dehydrated and felt nauseous. I would have a headache, and then the headache would go away. It would come back, and then it would go away again.

Throughout my run, all these little stupid things happened, but on this day, I experienced a pivotal moment: I talked to myself in anger as I powered through the annoying symptoms. I told myself, "You don't know discomfort. You don't know pain. You don't even have the faintest idea what it feels like to be challenged." I knew my mom was facing mortality, and here I was feeling sorry for myself because I was tired and dizzy.

I pressed forward with sweat and tears streaming down my face because I did not believe anything could be worse than fighting for your life and knowing you had a predetermined outcome. My mom was doing just that, and I was wallowing in my pit of despair. Her situation made mine feel so much less important. It didn't make it less real, and it didn't make my struggle any different; I just felt more compelled to overcome it. *I suddenly felt I had a choice.*

Mom was dying; she was fighting through chemo and chemo was killing her. The cancer was killing her. It was all taking her, and it made me realize how much control I had over my situation and my thoughts around my health. It made me realize how much control my father had over being diabetic and managing his lifestyle choices. It gave me a zero-tolerance mindset when it came to taking care of myself.

Though I didn't realize it at the time, having these insights was a critical moment for me as both an individual and as the transformational health coach I'd later become. I felt the urgency to step outside the story I was telling over and over. I had been telling the story of POTS repeatedly. When people asked me how things were going, I felt like I was on a soap opera. My story always revolved around my health.

I was tired of my story. I didn't need to talk about my situation, the state of my health, or the moment of dizziness that just passed. No one needed to know, and, quite frankly, no one cared. I finally became fed up with hearing myself tell that story over and over again, in my head and when talking to others.

Instead, I started searching for a different one.

I found it by delving into personal growth: podcasts, interviews, and educational shows. After listening to Shawn Stevenson on *The Model Health Show* podcast, I thought, "This guy could help me," so I reached out to set up a meeting with him. At the time, he was still doing one-on-one consulting, so I felt very grateful to have the opportunity.

In the months leading up to my visit to St. Louis, I wanted to walk in his door and have it all together. I wanted him to be proud that his influence was powerful. I listened to every single one of his podcast episodes before I went. I probably purchased everything he ever recommended, including Earthing sheets, Mountain Valley water delivery, and medicinal mushrooms. I implemented so many new detailed health-building activities in my life because of his trusted recommendations. By the time I walked in his door that day, I felt I had accomplished so much. I was going to him to find answers, but the answers were presenting themselves to me along the way. I had already made so many changes to my body and life that all of those seemingly "little" things had added up to *big* changes.

Remember how I referred to "my POTS" – how it owned me? It still did.

The first thing Shawn told me coincided with where my mindset was heading, which was away from the powerful story I was living. He explained to me that in my preliminary interview process, I had written the words "my POTS" repeatedly. I used other descriptive phrases of ownership as well, which led him to say, "You have it [POTS] written all over."

My first thought was, "Ugh, that's not who I am!" It was the first real smack of awareness in the face; I was telling my story as if POTS was me. It defined me even in writing.

Shawn asked me, "Why do you think this diagnosis happened?"

I said, "I think it happened for me, not to me. It made me who I am." I believe I had to go through the experience to see life through a different lens. What's crazy is I had not had this perception before, even after my meltdown with Mom. It became clear, at that very moment, what I had been doing to myself by accepting that negative story as my truth. It was the most eye-opening experience to sit with him and hear myself say the things I was already coming to realize. This meeting was another incredible turning point in my life. My gratitude to Shawn and the work that he does, the education he provides to the world, and his dedication to serving others is incalculable.

It was liberating to say, "I *can* change my story." Somehow, not only permitting myself to move on but also having someone else objectively point out his observations, was the "click" I needed. I had come to a place of being fed-up, which was a positive point in my journey.

DECIDING TO TRULY HEAL

Once I decided POTS was not my story anymore, I was very mindful of how often I used the term in my daily life and how often I called it mine. I was mindful of how often I talked to it in my mind and how often the symptoms would occur. I started to talk myself out of them. I began to deny and ignore them.

For example, when people would ask how I was doing, I reported I was great, even if I wasn't feeling 100 percent. It was better than the alternative of complaining.

When I would be in the middle of a workout and feel that rush of darkness come over me, I would casually sip my electrolytes, make sure I was sitting down,

54

sometimes go to the bathroom and splash some water and take a few deep breaths, but I would just get back to it when I knew I was *safe*. I didn't freak out or make it more real by focusing on the symptoms. I shifted my mindset into one of "*I got this. Nothing is new, this is how my body rolls and I know I can get past this moment.*"

I abruptly disowned POTS. I walked out on the relationship without warning.

Before doing this, it was crazy how often I let defeating thoughts come into my mind. Just being aware cut the frequency of them in half. It was extremely hard to eliminate the "I have" or "my POTS" anytime I even tried to have a conversation. After all, when you are married to something for years, it's hard to give it up cold-turkey. Suddenly, there is a void you must fill with productive energy.

Coaching and speaking are where I began to put that energy.

I realized my suffering was not in vain. It was my journey. Going through this pain was not simply to feel sorry for myself but to help others in my life overcome their obstacles, deal with their losses, and have hope for regaining their health and happiness.

I decided it was important for me to share my story to help people learn to be their advocates and not define themselves by their diagnoses. When I finally made this mindset shift, everything changed for me.

After my meeting with Shawn, I had found a new fiery determination. My symptoms seemed less persistent...or was it my focus had shifted on to more desirable feelings? I believed in the prospect of my efforts in creating *real* change. I had just been going through the mechanical motions of my symptom management, but it hadn't dawned on me before that I was on my way to healing. I began to dig deeper.

In my discovery, I uncovered nutrient deficiencies, gut imbalances, food intolerances, and detox issues. This insight showed me the root cause of my symptoms, which allowed me to apply principles and habits to improve my overall health. I can remove the bandages and heal the wounds from the inside out. I continue to build my health today. I do this by committing daily to follow the critical steps described in the next chapters.

56

CHAPTER 3

CRITICAL STEPS TO OVERCOMING POTS

"Start by doing what's necessary; then do what's possible; and suddenly you are doing the impossible."

– Francis of Assisi

POTS can be viewed as a jigsaw puzzle: identifying patterns, trends, and pieces that, when combined, tell an otherwise-fragmented story. You wouldn't try to force a puzzle piece to fit in a place in which it is so obviously not the connection. Therefore, you would not spend a lot of energy in that area of the puzzle. However, after connecting some other pieces of the puzzle, that section may begin to take on shape and meaning. The same piece which was a misfit may suddenly create a clear image.

In the same way, a puzzle missing a piece leaves no clear picture at all. There will always be a hole in the space that could otherwise bring together the entire picture. You need that missing piece to solve the puzzle.

Throughout this book, you will find pieces of your POTS puzzle. You will explore ways to discover what may have caused POTS in *your* body. You will be able to go deeper than you ever have with any conventional medical doctors. But aside from seeking a root cause, what might be more important is finding solutions that offer you consistent relief of POTS symptoms.

Living life with POTS does not have to be a constant drag. You will learn the tools that relieve your symptoms also improve other areas of your functioning such as improved mood and emotional energy.

This POTS healing system was developed as a result of many years of implementation not just by me but by patients and other individuals dealing with POTS. It was born out of a place of being exhausted by life with POTS. When I began to see the consistencies in successful outcomes, I was able to identify the types of behavior and lifestyle habits these clients had adopted that crossed over with what I also knew to be true and effective. I also noticed that without some aspect of each step, there can be missing pieces to the puzzle of whole health.

We are going on a journey and at the destination you will come to understand:

- How to get clear on your role and responsibility in your health and be in charge of POTS
- How to improve your lifestyle in a way that will dramatically decrease POTS symptoms immediately
- How to find a tribe of supportive people who get it
- How to practice true resilience and never stop learning
- How to embrace gratitude and why it matters with POTS
- How to dismantle old stories that are holding you back and create powerful new stories that support healing

The steps are best done in order. It is also recommended to focus on each step one by one. You will be spreading out the implementation over time. However, some steps may be part of your entire journey and will be maintained for as long as they become part of your life essentials. Those practices will continue to develop in an ongoing way. You will stack the habits within each step until they all become part of your being.

When you attempt to perfect too many tools at once, statistically, you are lowering your odds for building a successful ongoing behavior. Take your time. The order of the steps are designed to offer the education and guidance you need for any potential quick relief and rapid wins. It took me years to learn, adopt, and then continuously apply these many techniques! The beauty is that you don't have to continue digging, setting yourself up for failure, or wasting your precious energy and time. The steps work.

There may be other tools you have developed that work for you. There is no need to set aside something that is currently bringing you relief. Also, this information is not a replacement for the recommendations of your practitioner or team of doctors. It is not a replacement for medical treatment and care. And it is certainly not a prompt to remove any prescription drug from your treatment plan with your doctor without medical supervision. It is simply for you to have all of the information and tools that you need to make educated choices for your body.

Imagine getting your life back! Being able to relax about going out to eat or not having to explain yourself when people question your food choices or why you aren't drinking. Being able to conjure up the energy to walk into a gym or take a jog around the block. What if you could stand long enough to watch a presentation or take a hot shower without becoming lightheaded? Perhaps you can talk on the phone and walk at the same time without losing your breath. What would it be like to have a regular size meal without getting a tummy ache? Or not having to get up six times in the night because your bladder decided to kick into gear.

These are the simple things that people with even mild POTS would celebrate. What does your ideal day look like? What are some of the things that would be worth celebrating when your body begins to work for you once again? These are all things you will be able to answer during your time on our journey.

HOW WILL LEARNING THESE TOOLS HELP YOU?

First, healing and/or living with a chronic condition is about shaking hands with your condition but not letting it pull you down. I don't mean to downplay how tough life can be with POTS. In learning to live in spite of POTS, you will gain awareness and the necessary distance to break free of the old story and look at the situation through a fresh view. My purpose here is not to tell you to forget your diagnosis; it's to let you know that this thing you have doesn't have to rule the roost. It's just part of life and the journey.

You'll also learn new ways to advocate for yourself and nourish your body and mind. When you divorce your diagnosis, the journey to better health does not simply come to an end; you continue to investigate. You may find, as I did, the value of functional medicine in solving your medical mystery and re-balancing your body. Functional medicine is making waves and bringing about the change that is so necessary for our current failing medical system. It gives us the ability to look at pieces of the puzzle that were inaccessible in previous years. I talk about this in more detail in chapter 4.

Perhaps most importantly, you'll learn how to answer the question, "How do I learn to live again?" In the coming chapters, I answer this question partly through my experience, my research and my success, and partly through the personal journeys and words of some of the people I've been lucky enough to work within my career.

YOU DON'T LOOK LIKE WHAT YOU ARE GOING THROUGH

"You don't look sick."

"Please tell me what sick looks like and I'll try to get it right next time!"

Many diagnoses do not change the way someone appears on the outside. The person may not look like what they have been through. Therefore, it is easy to pass judgment on the severity of their suffering.

A couple of years ago, I had surgery on my hamstring and hip. I was confined to a walker with a giant brace on my leg and a strap on my ankle tied to the back of my waistline. I would use the electric wheelchair when I would do my grocery shopping at Whole Foods.

I was treated differently. I was looked at differently. But I had a wheelchair. People could see something was wrong. With many diagnoses and chronic illnesses, such as POTS, it's not so evident. I am consistently interacting with patients who are minimized for their level of perceived trauma. One was shamed because of her resilience. If she handled it well, it must not have been that bad. Another was dismissed by her family who assumed she was faking it. How could she be falling apart on the inside but still look well on the outside?

What about the person who is seen as the Ironman athlete, in fabulous shape, but people always wondered about the little pager looking box she always had tucked into her workout pants? The respect level suddenly shifts when you realize she is a Type 1 diabetic fighting the balance of her blood sugar with her insulin administration all day, every day. POTS is a secondary factor in her condition. The young women who struggle with painful stomach pain and unpredictable responses to what they eat in any public social setting do their best to pretend everything is okay while they try to have a beer with their college-age friends do not emulate the vision of a sick person.

YOUR DIAGNOSIS IS NOT YOUR DESTINY!

My desire for you and for others who have fallen victim to hurdles in their health and well-being is for you to find hope and belief again and see the potential of living a happy, fulfilled life, in spite of the POTS card you've been dealt.

POTS doesn't have to be your identity any longer. This book is about discovering a new side of the person that you are. It also about re-discovering the person you once were.

This book is about turning your mess into your message. It's about turning what begins as a burden and finding the blessing in the situation. Finding your message and the blessing allows you to know better, then do better, and then help others to find that strength inside of themselves.

The day you decide to change your story because you just don't like it anymore marks the dawning of a new you. You can avoid the emotional cost and devastation the unhealthy relationship with the diagnosis brings through simple awareness and choice.

You are not your diagnosis. You are not POTS.

I hope this book inspires you to recognize your power again! Believe in yourself and your body, no matter how many hits come your way. It's not about dismissing the reality of health concerns or dishonoring disease and diagnosis; it's about finding your truth and deciding how to live your life in spite of the obstacles and *never giving up*.

In this chapter, you have been prepared for the upcoming steps and how to go about using them. The next chapter begins in a place where many are already struggling – discovering their role in their own health journey.

CHAPTER 4

DON'T LET THEM TELL YOU YOU'RE CRAZY

"Doctors won't make you healthy. Nutritionists won't make you slim. Teachers won't make you smart. Gurus won't make you calm. Mentors won't make you rich. Trainers won't make you fit. Ultimately, you have to take responsibility. Save yourself."

—Naval Ravikant

This chapter is written to help you position yourself in your healing process. How much of the duty is on you and how much do you rely on the "experts" to get you the answers and improvements in your health that you are passionately seeking? Self-advocacy, or supporting your ideas and backing some of your judgments, matters because, at the end of the day, you are the one who has to live in your body and only you can identify and define what that feels like. You know yourself better than anyone else could ever imagine. When a doctor dismisses a symptom because the complaint doesn't get validation from a blood test or he ignores your pleas for relief because he can't find the problem, it is up to you to continue the pursuit. Some doctors may be very validating but lack any action steps to take you back to feeling like your body is working as it should. Frequently, that means stepping outside into a different therapeutic setting.

It's romantic to believe the medical world is going to have all of the answers. But the idea they have your back and will be there to support and relentlessly pursue your relief is fantasy. It requires the blending of your intuition and body awareness with the doctor's recommendations. In my case, once a doctor gave me direction, I began making decisions based on my new label of POTS. I started to disconnect from my body. I didn't listen to it anymore. Instead, I listened to what the *white coat* told me. Early on in my experiences with POTS, this set me on a path of treating each of my symptoms separately instead of looking for the root cause and addressing it.

The doctors do not have all of the power, especially if you do not give it to them. Take back some of that power and believe in yourself. Medicine can supply many of the missing pieces to your puzzle and give you the information you need to understand the dynamics of what your body and mind are dealing with. Once you have that diagnosis, you can proceed with educated decisions, but you are still in charge of your body.

I hear stories all of the time about the doctor that just wanted to give you pills or he blew you off, citing nothing was wrong with you and it must be psychological, not physical. Then I also hear the patient that puts full faith in their doctor and won't do a single thing outside of their doctor's direction. If the patient asks the doctor a question and the doctor says no, they take that word as some kind of world truth. They don't ever question their judgment.

TAKING CHARGE OF YOUR HEALTH HISTORY

When you know something is wrong but you can't get anyone to help you find the answers, it is very frustrating. After a while, you've started to think you are going crazy because there may be no quick justification for the symptoms you are experiencing. When you finally get a diagnosis, you might feel a sense of relief. A diagnosis may validate you. You have long felt like something is wrong, like you haven't been heard, or that doctors have dismissed you. A diagnosis substantiates your claims. It makes you feel like you aren't crazy after all.

At the same time, when you're diagnosed, you may also feel a conflicting emotion: fear.

The fear of not knowing and the fear of knowing are two conflicting emotions. On one hand, you wanted to know what caused your symptoms, but when you know better, often you feel obligated to *do* better – and that's not easy. You have to believe you can treat your symptoms, and you have to consider the change. But when you don't know, you can sit in your confusion and make excuses. For me, it was easy to blame everything on POTS.

It's hard to not fall victim to the debilitating mindset of a person with a diagnosis. That is what this book is all about. Why do some people become disabled in every aspect of their life after a critical health change, while others use the diagnosis as fuel to ignite their determination? They are listening to their intuition. They are talking themselves very carefully through each choice they make and where they position their energy.

When you decide to be your advocate, your journey doesn't end with the label; it begins with it. Remember: You are still in the driver's seat. You have to be.

I wasn't for a long time, and I had to make up for it later. In the beginning, going to the doctor was easy for me. My mom was like a walking encyclopedia when it came to my family's health timeline. She could tell you every detail of every appointment, every sickness, and every time I so much as had the flu. On top of that, she could tell you what year those instances happened. She knew every ounce of family history. When I would go to the specialist (in my case, neurosurgeon and neurologist, cardiologist, electrophysiologist, allergist, endocrinologist, general practitioner, etcetera) she was always there to sift through her mental Rolodex of my history. After all, she was there from the very beginning and never missed a beat. My mom was present for any significant appointment I had right up until she was diagnosed with bladder cancer. I was thirty-nine and still had Mom coming along for the ride.

No one preps us for the time when we sort of take over our health, let alone our parents' health. When I was on my own at my appointments, I knew nothing. I had no idea about my relatives' health history. I didn't even know my parents' details to the extent they ask you on an intake form. By deferring to my mother, I'd become dependent on someone else's memory about my health.

Later, when I became my dad's right-hand with his appointments and medical history, I witnessed the same situation. He had no idea about *any* of his family history and very little understanding of his health status. He would just smile and tell the doctor everything was great. I would simply think, "How can he just lie like that?" This blew my mind. It was as if he wanted to impress the doctor with his stellar health and positive attitude. Even basic details he got wrong. He would not recollect an important time related to a procedure, so he would give inaccurate details to the doctors who were relying on the patient to give them what they needed to best be of service. This situation was not just befuddling; it was dangerous.

Remember: When we give misinformation, we interrupt the prospect of getting the support we need.

I soon realized my dad didn't know how he felt. When dementia kicked in, he couldn't tell you what he ate for breakfast let alone how he was feeling last week. Yet working on his behalf, I could barely fill out his form, and some of the information I did complete was questionable for accuracy.

I did things differently for my mother. The day she was diagnosed, a dear friend suggested to me that I begin "a binder." Little did I realize how critical this binder would become in our process. I became her encyclopedia. Her binder was stuffed with every single medical record: every test result, scan, disc, report, event, prescription, and doctor's appointment. This binder became her health bible. We took it to all of her doctors and presented her case. Beginning with the

73

urologist that started the process, to the oncologist-gynecologist, the oncologist-hematologist, and the second opinion that was rendered after it was too late to take any further action.

This taught me the importance of creating my binder. I also recommend this to all of my clients. It is so important to be armed with your medical records *and* a full understanding of your symptoms and issues.

WHY SELF-ADVOCACY MATTERS

When I saw my orthopedic surgeon about a tear in my hip labrum, I was complaining of pain on my backside, deep in my rear muscles. We scheduled my hip surgery, but the week before when I went in for the pre-op meeting, I drilled the doctor, asking him how the hip repair was possibly going to fix the pain in my hamstring area. Hip injuries do create pain in various areas, but I wasn't convinced this was going to fix my problem.

He proceeded to ask me various questions about my hamstring pain. Confused and in agreement with me, he pulled up the DISC of my actual MRI and reviewed my hamstring area. In plain sight, there it was. I had a full hamstring avulsion, which is very uncommon in someone with my activity level and mostly seen in athletics, football, hockey, or sprint runners.

The hip MRI was done on my hip. The report was written on my hip. The hamstring injury was sitting on that same scan and had I not persisted in my concerns, I would have had a surgery that would not have brought me relief. Instead, I was able to have both procedures at the same time, cutting my recovery time in half. I also only had one deductible and one hospital bill. It was worth being belligerent to get the answer to my question.

THE BINDER

Medical records are a big deal and need to be at your fingertips. Keeping these records handy and understanding trends in your health are important to be your advocate. But where do you get those records?

Technically, your physicians create the files that contain your medical records, but the actual records and results are based on the findings of the patient. Their office established the record; therefore, the physical medical record belongs to the provider.

By law, a healthcare facility is required to maintain the medical record of each patient. The facility is extended the burden to prevent damage, loss, unauthorized use or alteration. However, the information gathered *within* the record belongs to the patient. As a patient, you are entitled to a *copy* of the record but not the original.

You may request to review or receive a copy of your record but may be subjected to a charge for the copy. The fees vary state to state. (For more information, visit the following Health and Human Services (HHS) site https://www.hhs.gov/hipaa/for-individuals/medical-records/index.html.

You may be familiar with the HIPAA (Health Insurance Portability and Accountability Act of 1996) rule, as you sign a form related to it for every doctor you may see. Many of us don't know what it entails. You can review the HIPAA Privacy Rule at HHS. It states: "The HIPAA Privacy Rule grants patients or their representatives the right to receive, inspect and review their health information, including medical and bill records, on-demand." (https://www.hhs.gov/hipaa/for-professionals/privacy/index.html).

By law, you are entitled to your health material. However, countless people are unaware of their legal right to access their records. Many won't even seek to obtain a copy and will just go by that random phone call from the doctor's office citing that "your blood results are normal." This isn't good enough. To know your trends and you need to know what "normal" looks like for you, which means you need copies of your blood work, writeups and other records. You need these for your binder, which I'll describe more below.

I can't emphasize this enough: *always request a copy of your medical records.* Fortunately, this is easier now than ever before. Access to electronic medical records and patient portals has made the record-keeping process even more efficient. Many hospitals and blood labs offer online access to test results and health records. If you are dealing with repeated labs, for instance, some portals will show you the history and past results in a snapshot, making it easier for you to view trends.

For keeping a medical records binder, I print these documents immediately. While the online tool is

77

great, you are often subjected to various doctors with multiple portals. You may seek various opinions out of different hospital systems that can't communicate. The binder is a physical tool you may carry with you to *any* doctor's appointment, giving them handy access to all of your results.

When you are seeking an additional opinion or attending another specialist, having the information at your fingertips is golden. Every doctor to whom I have presented the binder – my own, or my clients', or my family members' – is grateful and impressed by the patient's interest. I believe doctors also treat you with a little more respect. You present yourself as someone more educated about the system. You're not a victim following blindly with the rest of the herd.

Exercise: Preparing Your Binder

Once you get copies of your records, how do you prepare your binder? Here's how I do it, for myself and clients:

1. Set up your online access to all hospitals, clinics, and practitioners at which you have been seen, if they are offered.

2. If they do not offer electronic records, ask how you may access your health records and lab results. You may have to request them in writing and pay a fee.

3. Set up accounts with all blood and test labs you attend.

4. Review your history and obtain older records so that you may record a potential ongoing trend that was never identified.

5. Create your binder. The binder begins with basic tabs that may be divided by your doctor, lab results, various hospital records, testing performed, reports on results, and some pockets for CD images. This will look different for each individual depending on the depth and complexity of diagnosis.

6. A CD is important. Many doctors can see things on an actual scan that is not reflected in the report. The report is written up separately.

7. Every single time you attend a doctor's appointment, the record goes in the binder. Each test result you receive, the result goes in the

binder. Records of weight, symptoms, any type of journal entries can be kept here.

If a binder sounds like a pain to create, it is – but it can save you time, frustration, suffering, and sometimes even money. Remember: physicians can be your allies but they are fallible and they're often under a lot of pressure to see many patients in a day. It's up to you, in the small amount of time you have in the room with them, to help them see the big picture. As Dr. Maya Angelou said, "I learned a long time ago the wisest thing I could do is be on my side, be an advocate for myself and others like me."

DOCTORS AREN'T ALWAYS RIGHT

Have you ever met a doctor who seems confused by your symptoms?

In the early days of my diagnosis, no doctor ever knew what POTS was, though their egos were too big to admit that. Most doctors just looked at me and nodded their heads when I told them I had POTS, saying, "Oh yeah, I know what that is." Then they proceeded to do nothing consistent regarding treatment. One time, in the emergency room at Cleveland Clinic, I heard whispers outside of my curtain in triage. I peeked out from behind the curtain of my room and watched as two young nurses searched for POTS online. I could hear them asking, "What is it called?" Some of the nurses admitted they had not heard of POTS. They asked me about it. They were curious and wanted to know more.

At one point, I saw an endocrinologist out of Cleveland Clinic after I learned about my blood sugar imbalances. When I mentioned to him that I had POTS and thought there could be a relation between my blood sugar issues and the dehydration from POTS, he immediately said he knew what POTS was. First, he misinterpreted what I said. He thought I had Potts, which is a form of tuberculosis. When I clarified for him P-O-T-S, he wouldn't admit he didn't know what POTS was. I tried to explain to him how the heavy mineral imbalances and severe dehydration I experienced could somehow be related to my high blood-sugar readings, but he dismissed me, saying the connection was unlikely. He said my readings were not a big deal and to come back to him when I was diabetic.

I was not okay with that answer. I knew doctors didn't have time to help me. They weren't going to keep looking to try to find the missing piece to the puzzle. They were going to follow their protocols, their textbooks, their diagnoses, and the medications they lived by.

I walked away from that appointment extremely disappointed. After each doctor's visit, I walked away with disappointment or the feeling of having even less information than I had when I went in.

A few weeks later, I received a letter in the mail. It was from the endocrinologist at Cleveland Clinic. Dr. Patel not only admitted he was not familiar with POTS, but that he had done some research since I left. He reported that he did agree with me that there was a solid likelihood my dehydration was a factor in some of my blood sugar readings.

I remember being so incredibly proud. I walked around my work office like I had just hit the lottery. Dr. Patel took the time to write a letter to me, letting me know he could have been wrong. He was bold enough to swallow his pride and ego and give me a little bit of credibility. It reinforced my belief that I didn't have to rely on a doctor or someone with a different level of experience. I could trust my instincts.

That experience empowered me. Building a team and having support from physicians has made all the difference. Having different eyeballs analyzing your circumstances is going to bring the most successful outcome. But at the end of the day, you still need to know your stuff better than the doctors.

When you are empowered to take control of your health, you are educated, in charge, and learn everything there is to know about your role in healing your body. Imagine being able to fill out your health history with ease because it is all at your fingertips. It's not that this is something we all dream of doing, but it certainly makes you feel in control.

I succeeded in gaining the respect and help of doctors because I had become my own advocate, I knew my situation, and I was not letting someone tell me it didn't exist. Knowing that I had control over my symptoms and I knew my circumstances gave me more control to change them. It gave me more evidence of what I needed to do to feel better and disconnect from the label I'd been given.

Educating yourself on your tests is critical. Accuracy is not always guaranteed with doctors or anyone else. No one is perfect. When they are looking at results all day long between the rapid-fire schedule of patient after patient, the potential for error is great. The point is, having the binder is just half of the equation. You need to use it and stand up for yourself or your loved ones.

A powerful and unforgettable illustration of advocating for yourself or a loved one: after her full bladder removal, my mom's bladder surgeon reported there was no cancer in her lymph nodes. This came as a huge relief since the fear of chemo and/or radiation was my mom's biggest nightmare.

Within a day of the reassurance of her "clean" removal, a different hospital doctor working on her case came by before she was discharged. He casually advised she would follow-up with her surgeon regarding the lymph nodes and subsequent chemo that my mom had been promised was off of the table.

The moment the offices opened, I called and spoke with the surgeon. I had his backline number after a friend who knew him gave me an alternative number to reach his direct assistant. At this point, they knew me and were not going to leave me on hold. He picked up the phone and immediately maintained there was no cancer in my mom's lymph nodes. I was holding the report in my hands and calmly said, "You need to turn the page." When he flipped over to page two, he was forced to apologize when he realized he hadn't read the full report and was wrong all along. He had misdiagnosed the next steps and the stage of cancer.

He'd shifted the entire course of my mother's treatment because he simply missed turning the page to read the full report.

This is just one example of what it feels like to go into a health crisis uninformed and unprepared. When my mom was ill, I didn't know anything about traditional or non-traditional medicine or natural healing or any type of alternative or functional options. I didn't understand much about chemotherapy and what it did to the body. My family was in a moment of paralyzed fear. We made a lot of decisions at the discretion of the doctor. We were told what to do, and we did it like polite soldiers following orders.

Knowing what I know today, I would not have done things the same way, not for my mom and not for my family. I believe that my mom did a lot of things that we supported and encouraged her to do. I believe she did them for us.

My purpose here is not to tell you, "Don't trust doctors." You need them on your team. But you do need to bring your mind to the table, as well. Do not be afraid to speak up and ask as many questions as it takes to get the answers that bring you peace and certainty – at least as much certainty as is available to you.

Remember this quote from William Saroyan: "Doctors don't know everything. They understand matter, not spirit. And you and I live in the spirit."

IT'S ALL UP TO YOU

It is critical not to become overly confident in owning your health and diagnosis. You need the experts because we need to make consistency a priority even when we feel good. Traditional medicine performs lab work to establish trends. Traditional physicians look at how things are functioning at the moment. Reviewing
86

these labs continuously keeps you ahead of your health prospects. But not keeping up with regular check-ups, bloodwork, and physical exams can set you up for shocking diagnoses in the future. Traditional medicine has a time and a place.

When Mom was gone, I was in charge of my timeline. By this time, I had fired all of my doctors and was performing the testing myself since I had completed my schooling. Most people are not in a place to consider this. Therefore, it is necessary to be even more congruent with your doctors.

I had found my soulmate practitioner in functional medicine (more on this below).

My functional medicine doctor did not mess around with history. Functional medicine is sometimes casually called *root cause medicine*, as the goal is to seek what caused the break in the body's system. My doctor's intake system required over an hour to compile the lengthy background that, once complete, returns a summary of incredible data that points the arrow in the most prominent direction that will result in the biggest improvements. Boy, did this process open my eyes to my missing encyclopedia.

When it is you, your body, it is harder to be objective. When it came to me taking care of me, it was not as easy as I thought. The first time I found myself filling out my history for my functional medicine doctor, I was stumped. I didn't know my family history of cancer outside of my parents. I had no idea how old I was when I had my first round of antibiotics. I knew I inhaled them through my teenage and young adult years, but I had lost count of the frequency.

As for my history of physicians' visits... somewhere along the way, I had adopted a mindset of my traditional doctors failing me. I was stubborn. I hadn't been to a specialist or general practitioner in years. I refused to routinely go to anyone, except for my gynecologist and my orthopedic who maintained my aging knees.

However, I run my blood work, I listen to my body, and I eat the foods that help me to thrive. When you begin to own your health, you keep things in order. You make a log of appointments, you keep track of dates, diagnoses, scans, and tests. You watch your trends. If you don't, they become problems before you realize it.

After my dad died in 2017, my sister and I were cleaning the last of the boxes from my childhood home. In the boxes, I found medical records and blood tests on both Mom and Dad. I was shocked to see Mom and Dad *both* had diabetes trends that went back fifteen years. My mother's cholesterol issues had started years ago and my father's diabetes and blood pressure had been ongoing for years before the treatment started. *Who knew?*

This was information I would have loved to have known. Had I known about their trends – had *they* known about them – perhaps the progressions of their diseases could have been slowed through behavioral change or medications.

Staying on top of your routine testing and tracking your trends will set you up for success in the future, in spite of POTS or any other diagnosis. The more you know, the more power you have to your health.

THE POWER OF WORDS: THE NOCEBO EFFECT

Patients beware: do not underestimate the power of words from a person with perceived authority like a doctor. You must be aware of how to mitigate the effects of talking to many doctors as their language can send you in many different directions.

A nocebo effect is the induction of a symptom perceived as negative by a fake treatment or the suggestion of negative expectations. A nocebo response is a negative symptom induced by the patient's negative expectations and/or by negative suggestions from clinical staff in the absence of any treatment. Essentially, it means that if a patient is warned of side effects, they are often more likely to experience them.

For instance, one study asked two groups of patients to participate in a flexibility test. One group was warned of the possible pain associated with the movement. The other was told nothing. The group warned of the pain reported significantly higher levels of pain, despite enduring the same procedure.

I experienced both of these during the POTS diagnosis adventure. First, when my doctor told me I was simply "out of shape," I decided if I wasn't in any danger, what harm would it be to continue to be active even if I was breathless and on the verge of fainting? I endured the hot runs, the gym fatigue, and the dizziness.

90

I knew something was not right, but I assumed the discomfort was my normal, so I pushed through it. My doctor had said I was deconditioned, and I never wanted to feel this way again, so I ignored my fears and physical debilitation and pushed through.

On the flip side, when I was told I had arrhythmia and witnessed the change in blood pressure and heart rate, I immediately switched gears. I was validated in believing something was wrong. I knew I wasn't crazy! Now it was "confirmed" by an ER doctor that I was not "normal." It was sort of a relief, but I quickly fell into the fear of harming myself if I was overexerted, even though clearly what I had been doing for exercise was helping me.

The nocebo effect was powerful for me. Maybe you've experienced it yourself. When a doctor tells you that you will need medication for the rest of your life to maintain the stability of symptoms, you believe it regardless of the circumstances and your denial.

A doctor's words can have a powerful impact on a patient. Words are tools doctors should be educated on how to use, but as patients, we don't have much control over that. All you can control is your response.

You must beware of the potential impact of a doctor's words. While nothing a doctor advises should be initially ignored, you must sift through the facts and the opinion and separate them from each other. Remember, medicine is referred to as a practice for a reason. It is consistently changing, and no two doctors will have the same experience, knowledge, or opinions about it.

Imagine a doctor that has been in practice for over twenty years and goes to his office day by day, seeing similar types of cases day in and day out. Over time, what is the likelihood his recommendations become somewhat impersonal? Does he have the education of new studies? Is he proactively keeping up with medical discoveries or is he solely relying on his pharmaceutical representatives to teach him why their new drug should be prescribed to all of his patients? He doesn't know what he doesn't know.

I had several doctors. Some were very matter-of-fact: "It is what it is." Others almost catered to the diagnosis. For example, an electrophysiologist doctor gave me a book on the autonomic nervous system. Essentially, he wanted me to understand the basic principles of why people faint. His suggestion was both good and bad for me. The book he gave me taught me details about my body's process when I got dizzy or experienced headaches or nausea. I knew what I needed at that moment to "fix" the symptom. Most often, it was salt, water, or some sort of medication. The bad part of the book? It gave me detail into my body's process, which was almost too much information. I started to obsess over every little move, and I described in detail in my mind what I imagined was happening each time a symptom would appear.

Having too much information, especially from an authority figure like a doctor, may prompt you to self-diagnose. It can bring on additional perceived limitations. The information may cause you to create new stories since you may relate to the detail in a way that you begin to believe it's all hopeless.

Another doctor was fascinated by my presentation. I was like a circus act. He would place the heart-rate device on my finger. I would go from a sit to a stand and watch the number climb quickly to over 130 bpm when I hadn't even taken a step. I remember his wide-eyed response as he confirmed immediately that this was *not* an allergy. He said he wouldn't even test me for allergies because it would be dangerous to give me epinephrine. Another form of instilled fear is when a doctor appears freaked out by your symptoms!

INTEGRATIVE AND FUNCTIONAL MEDICINE

As I mentioned earlier, I got to a point where eventually I fired most of my doctors when I realized they were not looking at me, but rather as a cookie-cutter patient rolling through a factory. When I decided to be the CEO of my health, I researched, listened to podcasts, and enrolled myself in physiology and nutrition courses. I began to learn how food is used for medicine, and through this exploration, I discovered integrative medicine, functional medicine, and functional diagnostics.

The reference to integrative and functional medicine is often used interchangeably. While there are some distinctions, I don't see them being one better than the other. You can probably find a ton of crossover and people arguing for their differences for the sake of conflict.

Both look at discovering the root cause of a disease or diagnosis. Both take into account the lifestyle of a patient. Both treat the individual rather than the disease.

Functional attempts to find the underlying cause of a person's symptoms. Functional medicine uses lab analysis and non-conventional labs (labs that are not traditional in conventional medicine settings) that may expose various nutrient deficiencies, gut vulnerability, hormone imbalances, or toxic metals. All of these aspects of a person's health maybe a piece of the puzzle that may help identify the origin of an individual's health problems.

Functional doctors may use supplements and medications as necessary but they also focus on lifestyle factors that contribute to whole health such as sleep, stress, diet, exercise, and meditation.

Integrative medicine may have additional natural health features such as acupuncture, chiropractic, massage, nutritional coaching, etcetera. Some take into account many approaches to healing and combines them into a one-stop designed to create a custom package for the patient.

I love this analogy used by Chris Kresser: "If you have a rock in your shoe, you could take ibuprofen and that would help relieve the pain. You could also just take your shoe off and dump out the rock. Conventional medicine is prescribing the ibuprofen for that proverbial rock in the shoe." [3].

In my case, I felt that traditional medicine was masking my symptoms. Integrative medicine was looking for the cause of my symptoms. It addressed the *whole* person, not just the part.

I encourage my coaching clients to consider integrative medicine because it addresses POTS and the ANS and what went wrong to create the syndrome. But it does not give life to POTS in the way conventional medicine does. When you are working with a functional doctor, they are going to look at all aspects of your lifestyle. They're not simply attaching the complaint (symptom) to a medication (band-aid). The functional practitioner is going to dig deeper to find what could be causing the symptom.

If you are hoping to get off of some of your drug therapies, this approach is particularly helpful. *Conventional medicine may assign a lifelong prescription to your diagnosis. Functional or integrative medicine is more likely to help you avoid the need for unnecessary medications.*

As implied by the title of this chapter, I believe there are a time and a place for both conventional medicine and medication *and* functional medicine. The conventional model, for example, is exceptional for acute care and emergency medicine. I would certainly not go to an integrative doctor if I have just broken a bone or if I need stitches. But if you have an ongoing condition and you want to get to its root cause rather than treating symptoms as they come up, functional medicine can be a life-changer.

RESPECTING BOTH SIDES OF MEDICINE

Respecting the various sides of medicine – traditional, integrative, functional, and alternative therapies – and considering that each may contribute to your highest good will allow for you to examine options.

Knowing your options strengthens you and allows you to make your choices about your health. This matters a lot because everyone will have an opinion. Friends and family will have their point of view. You may have a peanut gallery of insignificant criticism that will disrupt your confidence. You may also know people who are purest in their thinking. They have an absolute way and no other viewpoint is entertained.

While my experiences with conventional medicine brought about very little effective change, the experience was a connection on my various trains to wellness. I needed to know and get what I learned from each doctor with whom I had an exchange. I got a little something from each of them: a book that ultimately empowered me; a misdiagnosis of being unfit, which drove me to work out; a direction to eat salt, which later led me to focus on my mineral balance; and a nudge to watch my sugar, which led me to discover my adrenal and liver issues and avoid becoming a diabetic. Nothing was without value.

One more note about conventional medication: it can be very meaningful in various diagnoses. While I don't believe pharmaceuticals were developed to be lifelong in their foundation, they often create a bridge to better health. In many cases, such as Type 1 Diabetes, medication may be lifesaving. Understanding how to manage medication and supply your body with the potentially depleted nutrients from pharmaceutical drugs can allow you to benefit tangibly from both sides of medicine.

Most of my clients come in with some variation of the same story. The doctors have dismissed their symptoms or only offered medication therapies and had no interest in finding the origin of POTS.

They have been reading and researching and finding little consistency and a lot of medication recommendations. They are struggling to maintain hope that they will once again feel normal. It is impossible to get people to understand what they are feeling since they often appear just fine on the outside.

This is why I begin with self-advocacy. It squashes the notion that the doctors are going to be driving the healing process and helps them to take responsibility for themselves. Once this mindset is set into motion, they can move on to how they will take the wheel and use their resources and the doctors' expertise to support their case.

IMPORTANT TESTING FOR POTS

When I was diagnosed with POTS, I didn't test for many things until years after I discovered their powerful significance. What's ironic is traditional labs for POTS are very *normal*. This is part of the anomaly that is POTS. A complete blood count would often not even reveal the dehydration or low blood volume associated with POTS. Standard labs in the hospital will mostly reveal nothing. If the doctor doesn't measure blood pressure and pulse in the lying, sitting, *and* standing position, he may never see anything odd.

Imagine my incredible interest when I learned the role that hormones played in POTS symptoms. How adrenals are impacted in a person with POTS symptoms is worthy of note. What key nutrients may be missing?

I often recommend the following tests to be considered when initially diagnosed with POTS:

- Cortisol Awakening Response and Rhythm Test: a saliva test which helps to establish a circadian rhythm disruption pattern for both cortisol and melatonin.

- Nutrient Evaluation: is the person's body effectively utilizing and producing key minerals and vitamins that support all of the workings of the body? Most often both blood and urine are measured.

- Gut Check: a fecal test that helps rule out any parasite, fungus, bacterial infections, as well as reveals how well the body is digesting and absorbing nutrients.

- Thyroid Markers: conventional measures TSH – Functional reveals T3, T4, Reverse T3, etcetera.

- Blood Sugar (fasting, A1C, and insulin): establishes if there is any insulin resistance.

Exercise: The Self-Advocate Checklist

- *Find your doctors.*

101

How do you know if a doctor is right for you? Do your homework. Look at the reviews of the doctor and their staff. Beware of the peanut gallery offering you the "best doctor" without looking into it for yourself. Everyone thinks they have the best doctor and it is very personal; what's best for you is measured by you. For information on functional medicine doctors in your area, you can use the Institute for Functional Medicine website at https://www.ifm.org/find-a-practitioner/

- *Build your binder*
  Use the guidelines in this chapter and bring it to any appointment you may have.

- *Create a journal of symptoms, questions for the doctor, and timelines*
  It is easy to forget things when you are at the appointment. If you have a list of written questions, you will make sure you cover your concerns. Knowing your symptoms and anything that may be connected (e.g. stress and stomach pain) is helpful for the doctor to do a thorough assessment.

- *Bring your "person"*
Having a third party present in your appointments is critical to objectivity. When you bring your advocate, that person is representing you in a sense. They are there to be your second set of ears. They may have questions that don't dawn on you at the moment. Your person is an extension of you.

- *Build your library*
With the information at our fingertips today, bewilderment is a choice. When we know better, we should do better. Figure out the optimal way you tend to learn and embrace that. For example, I am an auditory learner. I enjoy audio podcasts, audiobooks, and listening to interviews and inspiring talks. However, I am also visual and appreciate a good old hard-copy book. So I order both. I listen to the book on Audible.com and I purchase the book to highlight and use it as a resource. If you are a reader, an audio learner, or even do best in an educational setting, cling to whichever one motivates the most learning.

- *Realize that it may take a team*

Often complex diagnoses require a variety of doctors. POTS requires a team. Believing in each one of them is crucial. Having a rapport with each doctor will allow you to get the most from the relationship. As we have demonstrated, doctors do not know everything so having faith in their ability and commitment to helping you will improve your experience. The doctor's experience should not be a central stressor. Encouraging collaboration among your team will bring about possibilities for a better outcome. Most doctors address their "specialty" or their "part" of the body. They don't treat it as a system. Partnership, especially among functional practitioners and the patient, will bring about a systemic support structure.

In conclusion, you are the president of your own body. You hire your team and your doctors work for you. While their role is clear in the identification of the many puzzle pieces that make up POTS, you will be the person taking the action as revealed in the next chapters.

CHAPTER 5

DON'T THINK ABOUT IT, JUST DO IT – NUTRITION AND DIETARY PRINCIPLES

"Take care of your body. It's the only place you have to live."
—Jim Rohn

Most people think they are healthy if they are solely living in the absence of disease. Wellness encompasses physical, mental, social, and spiritual aspects of being. According to Marketdata Enterprises, people spend over $60 billion a year on diet and weight-loss products [4]. But when it comes to being healthy, the important ingredients extend beyond food. If you read anything related to wellness, you would understand

105

how important and underappreciated nutrition, exercise, sleep, connection and stress management is to overall health. However, when you are being delivered the news of POTS or any other diagnosis, there are likely no dietary and lifestyle conversations happening in the conventional medical setting.

Nutrition was the biggest needle-mover in my journey. When I changed my nutrition, eliminating sugar, processed foods, excessive carbs, and alcohol, my body began to heal itself. When my body became more balanced, my need for medications changed. But before we talk about getting off medications, let's talk about what food and nutrition can do to your body. I'll use myself as an example.

Before my formal POTS diagnosis, as well months after, I had started to notice a severe sensitivity to many foods that I could previously eat without any dramatic effect. Suddenly, I was feeling nauseous or sick to my stomach after eating sugar. Many superfoods that have powerful antioxidants would cause me to have diarrhea. Dehydration was the dreaded fear with POTS, so anything that upset my stomach was off-limits. The association between food and my symptoms was clear.

106

Any food that did not show as clear a cause and effect, I erred on the side of caution and removed it from my diet altogether. People used to tell me, "You are so disciplined." I responded, "No, I am deathly afraid. There's a difference."

Fortunately, making *do eat* and *don't eat* lists of foods was simple in my case; my body's responses were so obvious that it was somewhat easy to avoid foods that would do me harm. It was like a night in college where you may have had one (or several) too many shots of tequila. You spent that night and most of the next day sick as a dog. You swear to yourself you will never drink tequila again. Of course, you know the direct effect of too much tequila equating violent illness. Overdoing tequila typically results in such a painful experience that you promise yourself you will never have that feeling again. This association between an identified trigger and a physical response can go on for years, even a lifetime.

Unfortunately, for most people, avoidance is not quite as easy with food, unless you are outright food-poisoned. We don't often feel the effects of how food may bother us, or if we do, we don't know which food it may have been. If you went to McDonald's and had a

Big Mac, you may get a tummy ache – or not. But if you ate that same Big Mac and you immediately observed a six-inch expansion of your right thigh, you may reconsider Big Macs in the future. This is an example of the "Pinocchio effect," as one of my favorite podcast hostesses, Elizabeth Benton, so humorously puts it. We aren't usually this "lucky" with food. Our noses don't grow each time we eat something our body does not like. We don't feel the inflammatory response our body experiences on the inside.

In my case, the correlations were often very clear. That is not always true for everyone. Most people will need to be their "body detective" to match up what may appear to be unrelated symptoms. An example of something obvious might be when I would have stomach pain and diarrhea immediately after consuming a shake mix my friend recommended. Something not as obvious may be feeling extreme fatigue the day after I consumed a glass of wine or dessert. I might not as quickly make this connection. Until you are paying attention, the signals are easy to ignore.

When a client enters their highway to health, it is standard in my practice to consider an elimination diet or

108

detox of sorts. Eliminating various inflammatory foods, stimulants, typical gut irritants, or hormone-rich foods can help to identify some of these food and symptom parallels.

Often clients will report that "gluten doesn't bother me." And that is often outwardly true. They may not feel an immediate response when they remove gluten from their diet. What they don't realize is the impact gluten may be having on their brains. Or they can't imagine that the issues they see on their skin may not be directly associated with that bread they keep eating. Add to that the fact that they've often stopped paying attention altogether. When you are living in an unhealthy body, often unknowingly it becomes normal for you to feel bad after eating. You don't put two and two together. Just because tummy aches or fatigue is common for many people does not mean it should be the norm. As Alan Aragon said, "Every meal is a short-term investment in how you feel and perform, a mid-term investment in how you look, and a long term investment in your freedom from disease."

NUTRIENT DEFICIENCIES AND POTS

Medications, which are often recommended to manage POTS, can also play a role in how the body reacts to food. When I was in a body that could not balance itself, my minerals were off and I was in a constant state of malnutrition. Little did I realize that this had so much to do with the medications I was on, combined with my previous poor diet.

Before I got strict with what I put in my body, I was a sauce queen. I dipped my food in everything but was particularly fond of ranch dressing. I ate fried foods, processed junk, starchy bread, and way too many sugary sweets. On top of the imperfect food choices, here are the medications I was taking that were commonly recommended for people with POTS:

- Diltiazem (Cartia XT) to patch my racing heart. I had no idea it was also depleting my vitamin D, which drives strong bones and teeth, hormone production, and supports the immune system.

- A beta-blocker, also for the heart, was sucking my CoQ10, melatonin, and chromium dry. These key nutrients are crucial. CoQ10 influences energy production, protects your heart and skeletal muscles, and also boosts the immune system. Melatonin is the sleep-regulating hormone that helps maintain your circadian rhythm, has antioxidant effects, and is anti-inflammatory. Chromium aids in blood sugar control and insulin utilization, while slowing the loss of calcium.

- Midodrine to kick my blood pressure up when it would drop too low, so with it came headaches and a loss of magnesium.

- Zofran (Ondansetron) to relieve my nausea, but this also contributed to the dehydration headaches I felt daily.

- Celebrex (Celecoxib) to keep my inflammation down. But it also depleted me of folic acid, iron, potassium, sodium, vitamin C, and Glutathione – the very things my body was lacking as a result of POTS. What came first, the horse or the cart? Vitamin C and glutathione are vital antioxidants.

- Oral contraception, which I had been on for most of my adult life. It was depleting my beta carotene, most of my B vitamins, folic acid, biotin, pantothenic acid, magnesium, zinc, tryptophan, and tyrosine. These various nutrients are responsible for energy production and utilization, metabolism, thyroid function, and the list goes on. Magnesium alone is responsible for over 300 enzymatic functions as well as gut motility, cellular hydration, relaxing smooth muscle tissue that dilutes your arteries, and reduction in C-reactive protein, which is an inflammatory marker. Needless to say, if you are low on magnesium, lots of things can get out of whack.

It's no wonder my body was falling apart in spite of my efforts to get back in harmony. While I was getting "healthier" in my nutrition, exercise and expert symptom management, I was falling apart on the inside. Thanks to this malnutrition and its effects, I was diagnosed pre-diabetic when I was the fittest and thin I had ever been. My liver enzymes were higher than normal and my antioxidants were non-existent, indicating my body was

112

not detoxing well. I was dramatically low on B vitamins and glutathione (the body's "master antioxidant" used by every cell and tissue). My gut flora was significantly out of balance. My cortisol, melatonin, and DHEA were depleted, as were most of my sex hormones.

Can you believe I thought this was normal? That this was going to be my new life? But there was a reason I'd accepted this situation for so long. When I asked a cardiologist how long I would take heart meds, he responded, "For the rest of your life." So, that is the story I took on as my truth. But I don't know any drugs that have had trials that have lasted a lifetime.

I was taking some of these drugs for close to four years. How do we know what the effect of the blocking or enhancing our body's natural processes is doing long term?

I weaned myself off of these medications over time. I do not recommend doing this without the support and consulting of your physician. More importantly, I shifted my mindset from fearing foods to focusing on feeding my cells with nutrient density. Now I try to eat the foods that have the "biggest bang for the buck," meaning foods with the most vitamins and minerals I can

113

find like leafy green vegetables in high quantities; colorful, non-starchy vegetables; clean-sourced, organic, pasture-raised lean proteins; wild-caught fish; nuts; seeds; healthy fats; and moderate fruits. I stay away from grains and heavy-carb foods that lack nutritional value. I stick with sweet potatoes, quinoa, or other starchy vegetable carbs on my higher-carb days.

It felt like a miracle. I had energy again, my sleep improved, the dizziness faded, and I was able to build muscle. As my body started to get the juice it needed, I could physically feel the improvements. This took time and education. I continued my nutrition training through some of these transitions so I was my own walking experiment lab. When you have a compromised gut, you can eat as many health foods as you like, but if you are not breaking down and absorbing them properly, the additional support of supplemental vitamins and minerals may be appropriate.

Today, I monitor my nutrients closely. I test my vitamins, minerals, gut bacteria, cortisol and melatonin levels, thyroid indicators, inflammatory markers, blood sugar patterns, along with standard complete blood count (CBC) testing to assess overall health. The difference

114

year over year is remarkable and I am happy to say I am not only nutritionally stabilized but also at optimal functioning on many levels.

As you evolve in the healing process, your body and mind change. It's part of the process and part of growth. My body changed. My lifestyle changed. My friendships changed. My career changed. I became a better person because of all of it. I love my new self, but it took a long time to be able to say that.

Lifestyle changes are an evolution. I began with switching my little fake sugar packet from the pink one to the yellow and finally, the green. That was my progress. Eventually, I mastered various areas of nutrition and switched my focus to quality. Before that, I had no idea what a GMO was nor why organic meant anything to me. I couldn't tell you what chemicals were in my skincare products until I decided to care what they were. These things take time. It's a marathon, not a sprint, so be patient with yourself if you are new to paying attention to the things you put into and on your body.

Here are some other pointers, which I'll talk about more later in this chapter:

- *Remember, it's not just about food*

  Getting healthier is also about how you manage your stress. It's about the quality of your sleep. How well do you move negative energy and release things from your life that are no longer serving you? How much are you moving your body?

- *Change your activity level*

  If you are active, make sure activity works within your body's needs. As with diet, this also requires practice and experimentation. Sometimes simply changing a routine or pattern is beneficial. Our bodies tend to get complacent and need to be shaken up a bit now and then. For example, if you only do cardio for exercise, throwing in some weight training can shift your metabolism back into gear.

- *Feel what works best for you*

  Try different things. Focus on sustainable habits. Work on balance that will allow you to make permanent changes. Quick-fix diets and overdoing it at the gym will only lead to burn out. Learning to change it up will give you more variability that will keep you engaged and allow for flexibility. Knowing that something may stop "working" is not a tragedy, it is an opportunity to look at jazzing up a routine and knowing that the adaptability will allow you to rotate through effective techniques continuously

- *Measure your progress. Know your numbers. Get tested.*
  We discussed working with a functional practitioner in chapter 4.

Before I started my journey with POTS and functional medicine, I used to think people don't generally change. We all have values and core principles by which we live. However, I grew to realize that we can add to these core values and principles. Positive change is an opportunity to discover the very best of yourself. People can and do change. Change is a reason for progress.

People tend to resist change. We are creatures of habit and our bodies fight for homeostasis. This means physiological changes like blood pressure, heart rate, or body temperature (that may result from exercise, for example) can be taxing on the body as it tries to get back to its happy place. Neurologically, our "primitive brain" is responsible for wiring habits. Routine habits we are familiar with make us feel good.

Your friends and family may not respond warmly at first to your changes. I found my food choices made people around me very uncomfortable. My exercise was teased as "obsessive." At the end of the day, you become a mirror for others and their discomfort is only the judgment they are placing on themselves. Perhaps they would like to eat better or they are questioning their fitness level. Sometimes, it is just that they are watching you grow and they simply feel left behind. Lead with compassion, but stick to your truth. This is your life, your body, and your experience. You will disappoint some people inevitably, but that's okay. It's not about you; it's about their self-reflection. Just like you can't get sick enough to help a sick person get well or you can't get poor enough to help poor people become prosperous, you cannot worry enough to prevent disappointing people.

Nutritional and lifestyle changes may seem hard at first, but living with dis-ease is an exhausting and
118

much harder burden to bear. The prefix "dis" means "not or none". Therefore, dis added to the beginning of the word ease changes it to mean *without ease*. Disease is a deviation from the normal structure of an organism. Making the changes is worth every ounce of struggle and becomes a great deal more effortless as you adapt to the cleaner way of living. Starting from a place of good health makes it a heck of a lot easier to overcome the hurdles life throws your way.

Food is your body's life fuel. Real food makes you stronger. When you measure your nutritional status, you can strategically manage your progress.

WHY NUTRITION MATTERS

Nutrition is a huge needle-mover for POTS and many other conditions because the root cause of what's happening in people's bodies is often not only one thing – it's a system of parts affected. One part runs off of another. There are numerous systems of the body which include digestive, circulatory, nervous, respiratory, and muscular. They all work together to perform crucial jobs to run your body. Your body is responsive to any little thing that may be "off" on the inside. That minor break in the system can cause a cascade of events that ultimately affect many parts of the body's structure. But nutrition can often be an obvious mechanism to repair that break. Here's how:

Food is information. The nutrients in the food you eat are essential for the growth, development, and maintenance of your body's functions. As you take in various fats, proteins, and carbohydrates, each macronutrient tells your body how to break it down and each serves a function to the health of your cells. Literally from the point of chewing your food, you are introducing it into your body so that it can become part of your DNA. Conversely, when you are taking in "fake food," your body doesn't recognize it as food at all. Fake food usually involves ingredients you cannot pronounce, chemicals that were not likely designed to be used by the human body, or food that has been put through a process that strips it of natural nutrients and replaces them with fillers, taste enhancers, and/or texture substances. Many processed foods may be addictive as they can stimulate the reward systems in the brain, similar to that of other abusive drugs like cocaine. [5].

120

Fake foods cause inflammation, which can lead to chronic illness. These foods have been altered and deconstructed from their natural form to enhance flavor and to extend shelf life. This can devastate the bacterial harmony in your gut. Imagine the internal pollution you are being exposed to when eating processed junk.

It's funny; when you begin healing POTS, you may not recognize how much dietary changes played a role because there are so many moving parts. Healing is a process and diet is part of that process. Nutritional changes can bring about immediate relief of symptoms to many conditions. The food you put in your body is directly impacting the state of your human cells. Other moving parts such as stress triggers, sleep improvements, eliminating common environmental threats, or quieting the noise in our minds that hold us back from healing will also be partly responsible for the improvements.

With POTS, so much has to do with sheer determination after a shift in the mindset. It takes both conviction and dedication to eliminate foods and change eating patterns. It is critical to stick with the nutritional changes long enough to see results. Relying on principles and routines will help to keep you on track.

When I coach clients, we spend a lot of time on principles that support health – learning them and sprinkling them into the daily routine. The basic principles I cover are hydration, healing and stabilizing foods, exercise, supplements, meditation, sleep, gratitude, mindfulness, identifying and changing the stories that dictate our belief systems, and journaling. Each area has its subset of principles, which I like to call the *Rules of Thumb*. These *Rules of Thumb* help to keep you focused on what matters to your health.

For example, often my clients will get in the weeds on a topic that is not at the core of the real problem. They may ask me a question like, "Is it okay if I eat carrots? Because I heard they have higher sugar." They focus on the downsides of this otherwise healthful choice. Meanwhile, they are not prepared with their meal options and still struggle to get through the day without running through the drive-through. Bottom line: I am not worried about the sugar content in a carrot if you haven't been consistent with the over-arching theme of eating a clean diet. Sticking with the consistent basics of nutrition is going to move the needle more than avoiding a serving of a root vegetable. What are the basics of a clean diet? Here's what I tell clients.

NUTRITION RULES OF THUMB

- Avoid added sugar and white carbs that quickly convert to sugar. (AKA simple carbohydrates like bread, pastries, pasta, rice.
- Avoid artificial sugars.
- Avoid gluten-containing foods. Even if you are not considered gluten sensitive, it can affect your skin, stomach and/or your brain. Also, watch your consumption of the "gluten-free" fad foods full of sugar and other processed flours.
- Avoid toxic oils like soybean, canola, vegetable, etcetera. Rather choose clean fats with stability such as avocado oil or coconut oil for heating and olive oil for salads.
- If you can't pronounce it, make sure you know what that ingredient is before you consider consuming it.

- If a recipe or product has more than five ingredients, you may want to seek an alternative.
- Eat plenty of veggies and keep your fiber high (seven to nine servings of veggies *per day*).
- Caffeine should be consumed in moderation. If you have to use caffeine to keep you functioning, there is something bigger happening.
- Dairy is considered inflammatory and can be problematic for many.
- Hydration is critical. The quality of water is just as important. Tap water can be contaminated with pharmaceutical drugs and heavy metals in some municipalities. Using a filter, at the very least, will help. A reverse osmosis water system is a great option. And, better yet, invest in glass bottled spring water from a clean source. Bottled water is assumed to be the better alternative, but often it is simply tap water. Dasani, owned by the Coca-Cola company, is a great example of tap water filtered and bottled. But the chemical BPA (Bisphenol A) found in plastic bottles and other unsuspecting places like grocery receipts is

known to disrupt the endocrine system. This means it can interfere with hormone systems in your body. It's not simply the water source, how it is bottled matters. [6][7]

All of the above are rules with broad application, intended to be easily applied and easy to remember. Of course, it's important to recognize that personalization with nutrition is critical. What works for some won't work for others. We have more bacteria in our bodies than we do DNA. Everyone's bacteria balance is different. What one person can tolerate may make another person feel terrible. Some "healthy" foods may not be "healthy" for everyone.

However, the Nutrition Rules of Thumb are true for most. The nutrient-poor and fake foods described earlier are only going to exaggerate an already chronic issue. Various conditions may have more specific principles and it is important to understand this. For example, someone with candida would not want to be eating fermented foods, but they are exceptionally good for many people's gut bacteria. Other examples of customizations you may need to make:

- A person with Hashimoto's might benefit from cooking certain vegetables versus eating them raw.

- A person with rheumatoid arthritis may do well to avoid the nightshade category of vegetables.

- Someone with IBD or Crohn's will digest differently than someone with a less vulnerable gut. For example, "roughage," or the indigestible fiber found in plant foods, is typically discouraged for these disease states but the need for fiber in the diet is crucial for the elimination of waste from the gut.

You get the picture. People vary. Nevertheless, most people want to know what other people are doing when they see some sort of success. "Oh, you lost fifteen pounds? How did you do it?" Then they try to follow the same thing and it doesn't work. Remember, each of us is unique. Don't set yourself up for failure.

Ketogenic diets are a great example of people jumping on a bandwagon of a diet that works if you are eating "clean keto." But it doesn't mean keto is a long-term solution or that the way people are practicing keto is safe. There are many dynamics to the keto diet than simply measuring ketones. Keto is a hot topic in nutrition today and has solid research to support its powerful impact on people with various conditions, especially that of the brain. Keto can aid in weight loss, at least in the short term. The problem with some keto practices is the quality of the fats that are chosen and the significant lack of vegetables and fiber recommended in the diet. Loading up on hormone- and antibiotic-flooded fatty meats is not the same as eating an organic grass-fed cut of beef or a pasture-raised chicken. The old saying goes, "You are what you eat," but truly, your cells are made up of what you eat eats. Those hormones transfer to you.

In my years of working with clients, changing and tailoring their nutrition is the quickest way to get them to begin feeling better, even if just a little. If you're getting started, this may look like an elimination diet, a detox period, or simply cleaning up your food choices at first. A great place to start is with awareness. When we do more without awareness, we get into a cycle of reacting. When we are aware, we pay attention to what's working and what's not. We pay attention to how we feel when we are making food choices. When simply going through the motions and eating mindlessly, it is easy to

127

disconnect from a particular symptom. For instance, if you get bloated quickly after eating, pinpointing what you ate that may be the culprit is going to be more clear when you take your time chewing and enjoying your food. Notice how your stomach feels before, during, and after your meal.

What follows are some steps to begin raising your awareness of your nutrition and food choices. Remember, adopting new lifestyle habits don't happen overnight. Begin with a goal of progress, not perfection. It's all relative to where you are beginning. Someone who eats generally clean may have a goal to eat more organics in their diet. That is their progress from an already-sophisticated eating style. Another may be accustomed to driving through a fast-food chain daily and needs to improve on this. Progress can be as simple as converting from McDonald's to Chipotle. It's respective to where the individual is on their health evolution.

STEPS TO IMPROVING YOUR NUTRITION AND FOOD LIFESTYLE

128

1. *Log what you eat for a few weeks – it will open your eyes. Wide.*

You can't fix what you don't know is broken. Using an app such as "Lose It" gives you visibility to the approximate amount of fats, proteins, and carbohydrates you are consuming which are further broken down into fiber and sugar. Most people have no idea how much sugar or simple carbohydrates they are eating. The app shows the breakout by the percentage of each macronutrient so it is easy to recognize where you may need more protein or if you are eating too many starchy or sugary carbohydrates. For example, the FDA's daily recommendation of fiber intake is twenty-five to thirty grams. However, dietary fiber intake among adults in the United States averages about fifteen grams per day. I saw a guy who was trying to gain weight and I could see by his logs he was eating (and drinking) the wrong foods to get there – including over 100 grams of sugar per day! People often don't recognize a deficit or surplus with the types of food they are eating; tracking your food with a visual app helps them to realize their pattern.

2. *Practice an elimination diet.*

Sometimes we don't know foods are bothersome to our body until we take a break from eating them. Commit to removing dairy, gluten, caffeine, processed foods, sugar, artificial sweeteners, eggs, and alcohol from your diet for at least three weeks. After three weeks, if you so choose, reintroduce each one slowly and wait three days between each. Tune in to what you feel with each type of food. You may journal what you notice physically during and/or after a meal. Do you experience stomach discomfort? Perhaps you feel sluggish? Are you energized and focused? You may find that some of these foods are best to leave out of your diet all together, but again, it's a progression. The goal is to develop a sustainable way of eating. You may also find a food sensitivity test will fast track this process.

3. *Learn about nutrition.*

Read books, listen to podcasting health shows, and watch webinars. Seek out the thought leaders in health. *Be careful to understand the motives behind all the information.* You must consider the motive of the author of an article, research study, or claim. For example, when the American Heart Association had its Heart-Check seal on cereals such as Trix, Cocoa Puffs, Lucky Charms, and French Toast Crunch, it might make you raise an eyebrow. It doesn't take a nutrition degree to know Trix cereal is not optimal fuel, but as consumers, we need to question this seemingly obvious dissonance. (Fortunately, I have seen this trend changing since these cereals were removed from the Heart-Check approved list. However, there are still many questionable items being supported.) When *JAMA* (*Journal of the American Medical Association*) exposed how the sugar industry-funded research in the 1960s and then paid researchers to downplay the risk of sugar and highlight the hazards of fat.[8] By the late 1980s, everything was fat-free, low fat, and fake fat – a trend that has landed us the sickest and most obese in American history. The point is, consider the source. Research the authors, companies, and websites that host the information, because, for every piece of information you read, you will find a conflicting message with the click of a button. When I first became a research girl, I did not only take courses, but I also made sure to cross-reference both conventional and "natural" or integrative models. I looked across the different approaches for consistency in the message. I read the original research, not just a blogger's impression of it. I experimented on myself by trying a variety of food combinations. I ate low-fat, low-carb, high protein. I tried high fat. I experimented with way-too-low carb. I used my instincts. Make sure you are asking questions and listening to your body, not jumping on diet trends that won't last. It's not one-size-fits-all, so if it's not working, it's time to try something else. The best judge of progress is your body and how you feel, and of course, knowing you're where your health numbers stand.

4. *Recognize that you aren't just what you eat: you are what "what you eat" eats, too.*

When I learned that in the United States, antibacterial use in food animals is estimated to account for eighty percent of the nation's total antibacterial consumption, I wondered how that translated to me. Not only does the use of antibiotics pass along and affect the human who is eating the animal in which it was administered, but the animal's actual stress hormones are also impactful to humans, according to the FDA. (Look here for more information: https://www.pnas.org/content/112/18/5649)

Who knew? I know I didn't.

Nor did I understand the importance of organic and non-GMO for eating foods free of pesticides, contaminants, and hormones.

5. *Utilize the EWG.org website.*

The Environmental Working Group provides wonderful information regarding clean products and the safest foods for us to consider. It's helpful to print out the wallet insert with the Dirty Dozen and Clean Fifteen for reference while you are grocery shopping. It is also a great resource for learning about GMOs and other dangerous

133

chemicals in our food and body care supply. The Dirty Dozen and Clean Fifteen are lists generated as a "Shopper's Guide to Pesticides in Produce™." They give you a ranking of the most popular fruits and vegetables and which have the most pesticide and herbicide contamination.

WHO AND WHAT IS BEHIND THE MARKETING OF FOODS?

Money.

The Global Wellness Economy Monitor reports that healthy eating, nutrition, and weight loss is a $702 billion industry. The moment a diet is the talk of the town, the food companies grab hold of it and begin the manipulation of marketing. Suddenly everything is "gluten-free," "keto-friendly," "Paleo," etcetera.

The problem with these pre-made foods is the gluten is replaced with other processed flours and sugar. Keto food can be dirty, or full of hormone and antibiotic-ridden meats, artificial sugars, and unhealthy oils. Paleo is often protein overkill if the person is misunderstanding the body's appropriate protein needs. Non-GMO doesn't mean safe and doesn't dismiss the significance of organic. Organic is even questionable as some of the "acceptable" ingredients in the organic labeled foods are subject to a biased board vote. E.g. Carrageenan, a thickening agent with controversial health implications, is considered satisfactory for use in organic products.

These label claims are even placed on foods that are void of the ingredient intentionally. For example, egg cartons and chicken packages have so many claims, your head will spin. Cage-free, pasture-raised, non-GMO, organic, antibiotic-free, hormone-free, you name it. If you notice, a little asterisk on the corner of the package will reveal that federal regulations prohibit the use of hormones in poultry. So, why make the claim to begin with?

If there is money to be made, the big food and big pharmaceutical companies will find a way to get into the game.

I was walking through Whole Foods the other day and picked up a bag of dark chocolate chips. The label touted the contents as a "no-sugar-added, vegan, non-GMO premium baking chip." I noticed a second bag

135

of these chips on the shelf right next to the first. Except this bag proclaimed "keto" chips. I looked at the ingredients and they were identical, word for word. This company was simply catering to the keto consumer, making it a selling point on the label.

This relabeling process happens all of the time in the pharmaceutical world. When a brand drug's patent expires, the generic is launched by other companies, in theory, at a lower cost to consumers. It didn't take long before the brand companies realized that to stay in the money, all they had to do was call their branded product by the generic name, slap on a new label or market it through another company, and continue to profit off of the drug. This was known as the "authorized generic."

Big food wants a piece of the action and will pay big to enter the space where the consumer is leaning. Parent companies are not required to put their names on labels so it isn't obvious who owns the product. When you pick up a product with claims of *homemade*, you may imagine a little family farmer handpicking our ingredients and a grandma in the kitchen baking with her fresh-picked apples, the delicious scent of cinnamon flooding the home. Even these companies can't resist the monetary perks.

Many of the clean, organic, small Mom-and-Pop companies just sell out because the big food companies make them an offer they cannot refuse and a promise of no disruption to their initial mission. Did you know that many of the organic companies with some of the most popular clean foods are owned by some of the largest processed food companies out there? [9] Over eighty percent of organic companies are now owned by sizable food corporations. Maybe we should start calling it "Big Organic."

Let's look at some fun facts:

Big Food and the "Big Organic Takeovers"

- Coca-Cola owns Odwalla, Honest Tea, Green Mountain Coffee, and Dasani water
- PepsiCo owns Naked Juice and Aquafina water
- M & M/Mars owns Seeds of Change organic seed company
- Kellogg owns Kashi, Bear Naked, Wholesome & Healthy, Morning Star Farms, and Gardenburger

- General Mills, a company whose CEO wrote a letter asking to have GMOs called "natural," owns Cascadia Farms, Lara Bars, Annie's, Food Should Taste Good, and Muir Glen
- White Wave owns Silk, Earthbound Farms, Horizon, So Delicious, and Organic Cow of Vermont
- Smucker's® owns RW Knudson's organic juice
- Hormel, a pro-GMO meat company, owns Applegate Farms
- Danone Group (Dannon) owns Stonyfield Organic Yogurt and Brown Cow

These are just a handful of examples that make you scratch your head and hope that the quality of the brands you once admired for their health mission stays true.

Fortunately, there are a few companies still standing independently. Below are some examples.

Organic Companies Still Left Standing Strong
- Amy's Kitchen
- Bob's Red Mill

- Cliff Bar: Luna
- Eden Foods
- Lundberg Family Farms
- Nature's Path: Country Choice Organic, Enviro-Kidz
- Organic Valley: Organic Prairie
- Pacific Natural Foods
- Springfield Creamery: Nancy's
- Traditional Medicinals
- Yogi Tea

SUPPLEMENT COMPANIES

Supplements are also at risk of selling (cashing) out. How about Nestle's purchase of supplement companies such as Garden of Life and Pure Encapsulations? Garden of Life was known as a leader in the natural products industry. Self-proclaimed fanatics about what goes into their products, they held a standard of real, healthy nutrients, clean from chemicals, and are connected to every source of ingredients and handling of their products. I remember years ago hearing the owner on a podcast and admiring the passion for what he was putting out into the world.

Pure Encapsulations is known for its *pure*, premium ingredients. They avoid artificial ingredients, dyes, allergens, and contaminants. They even carry hypoallergenic supplements.

Nestle, well-known for their chocolate, is also a major manufacturer of the largest source of Enteral feeding formulas, which are used primarily in hospital settings for people who require feeding from a tube. The first three ingredients of one of the formulas are water, corn syrup, and maltodextrin, which is a highly processed food additive made from corn, rice, potato starch, or wheat and is closely related to corn syrup solids.

Another reputable supplement company that can be found in your nearest Whole Foods Market or high-end supplement store, New Chapter, is now owned by Procter and Gamble.

This doesn't automatically mean the quality and standards of what began as a mission-driven health company will waver, but it is something to be aware of when you are using these products. Anytime I observe a
140

change in ownership, I pay attention to the quality control if I continue to use or recommend any of these products.

It's an advantage to be educated on the companies that manufacture the foods you choose to consume. We vote with our dollars and what companies we choose to support each day. It helps to feel good about the story behind the food on your plate.

SLEEP AND STRESS MATTER TOO

Two of the most overlooked and mishandled aspects of our health, in my opinion, are the importance of sleep and addressing the big fat stress bus most of us ride daily. In my old corporate world, the more hours you spent in the office, the late-night emails, and the more drama you visibly could carry on your shoulders, the more "successful" you were regarded.

According to a Consumer Reports survey (https://www.consumerreports.org/sleep/why-americans-cant-sleep/), twenty-seven percent of US adults reported having trouble falling or staying asleep most nights and a whopping sixty-eight percent admitted they wrestle with sleep at least one night a week.

Nearly ninety percent of visits to doctors are for stress-related problems. [10] While stress is a natural part of life, if your stress response does not get a break from constant triggering, it can cost you your health. Stress can affect most aspects of your body including the respiratory and cardiovascular systems, the reproductive system, digestion, immune system, and the muscular system.

THE MAGIC OF SLEEP

Ongoing sleep deficiency is linked to increased risk of heart disease, kidney disease, high blood pressure, diabetes, and stroke.

- In general, exercising regularly makes it easier to fall asleep and improves quality and soundness. However, exercising sporadically or right before bed can disrupt falling asleep. Tip: exercise in the earlier part of the day can improve sleep. If you only have the evening option, create an evening ritual to help you wind down such as an Epsom salt bath or journaling.

- Most healthy adults need seven to nine hours of sleep per night. Some individuals may function without drowsiness after as little as six, while others need ten hours to reach peak performance. Sleep is regulated by two processes: homeostatic and circadian rhythm processes. In POTS, these processes are disrupted and need extra support. It is critical to establish a consistent sleep pattern when diagnosed with POTS.

- A night of deprived sleep can create a rise in appetite as the hormone leptin (that tells your body you are satiated) is lower. Have you ever noticed feeling more cravings after a night of poor sleep? You can't seem to get enough snacks in? One night of poor sleep can result in a decrease in Leptin sensitivity and an increase in Ghrelin (the hunger hormone). As a result, there is an increase in appetite and can be associated with a higher body mass index. [11]

- Social Jet Lag can occur when you sleep in on the weekends. We are the only mammals willing to

143

delay sleep, but that doesn't mean it's okay. Try to keep your wake and sleep times consistent. Tip: hit the hay at approximately the same time each night and even on days when you can sleep in, consider keeping it within an hour of your normal wake time. In doing this, you are better off having a short power nap and keeping your circadian rhythm in check.

- Being awake for sixteen hours straight decreases your performance as much as a blood-alcohol level of .05 percent. The longer you go without sleep, the more evidence of a decline in cognition. [12]

- Blue light from your electronics disrupts the secretion of melatonin. Consider investing in blue light blocking glasses to protect your eyes in the early hours leading up to your sleep time. Tip: avoid electronics or install blue light blockers on your devices. You can also buy tiny blue light blocking stickers to cover electronic power lights, routers, appliances, and more. Using amber colored light bulbs to relax can be helpful as well.

- Create a sleep ritual to wind down before bed. Dim the lights, take an Epsom salt bath, journal, practice gratitude, spend time with your loved ones. Tip: give yourself an hour to end your day. Also, consider this time as a time for peace and reflection on the day. You may also plan your efforts for the next day so you don't wake up in disarray on how to begin your day. The way you start and end your day can be pivotal to your productivity.

- Keep the air between sixty-two to sixty-eight degrees to help adjust your body to its natural changes in temperature. Invest in quality sheets and sleepwear. Tip: the slightest change in temperature can impact your sleep quality. Sleeping on an uncomfortable bed or with restrictive clothing can be disruptive to your ZZZZ's. Body temperature decreases at night time and rises as you wake. Research has shown how heat can disturb the delicate balance in sleep and body temperature. [13]

- Make sure your pillow is keeping your neck in alignment with your spine. Neck pain and waking body aches can certainly keep you up at night. Try a pillow that conforms to the shape of the neck and keeps it from over flexing your chin towards your chest or extending back too far. Sleep disruption from awkward positions or other factors can also affect the reparative processes that take place while you sleep. [14]

Sleep is the bomb. It's when all of the magic happens. The brain detoxes during sleep through its cleansing system – the lymphatic system. During sleep, we consolidate memories, making short term memories into the long-term. Sleep is the time when our hormones are releasing, our tissues are rebuilding, our energy is restored, and our bodies release muscle tension. These body functions take a tremendous amount of energy and cannot be done in tandem with the daily activity in our lives.

Sleep is so crucial to health that sleep deprivation can be used as a weapon of debilitation. It has been used by the CIA for interrogation and has been considered to be an act of "torture". [15]

HOW TO CHANGE YOUR PERCEPTION AND RESPONSE TO STRESS

Research shows almost every bodily system can be affected by stress. It is estimated that up to ninety percent of all visits to primary care doctors are for stress relevant complaints. [16]

Stressors include things such as the obvious intensity of daily life, food sensitivities, nutrient deficiencies, some forms of intense exercise, hormonal imbalances, pathogens like bacteria, fungal overgrowth, or viruses. Even positive things (eustress) can be considered a stressor. Each one of these biological stressors impacts the body in different ways. It can be in the form of inflammation, homeostatic disruption, and/or changes in the body's fight or flight response by simple adrenaline from a state of excitement.

147

We've known about the negative effects of stress for almost thirty years. In 1983, Time Magazine featured a cover photo titled "STRESS!" and declared it the epidemic of the eighties. Can you imagine? Life seemed so much simpler back then, at least to my generation. I imagine today's title would be even more explosive. In essence, stress is a part of life that is not going to simply disappear. It's not realistic to think that we have a huge amount of control over the daily darts we tend to dodge in today's world.

What is controllable is our reactions to stressful situations and our ability to prepare for them. Every day, we are faced with challenges that demand the best of ourselves. Have you ever noticed sometimes your coping skills are excellent and you don't even break a sweat? Other times you can barely handle someone looking at you the wrong way.

The stress response triggers physiological responses such as a racing heart, breath changes, muscle contraction, an increase in blood sugar, a shut-down of hormones and the immune system. Your body recognizes the priority of fleeing from a life-threatening circumstance instead of diverting energy to the reproductive system or fighting an infection. POTS is classic for having a disruptive stress response. The body's preference is to stay in the sympathetic overdrive. Using the common example of our ancestors fleeing from a threat such as a tiger or lion, our body uses these responses as a protective mechanism. It can be beneficial in the short-term. But when the stress becomes chronic and lasts much longer than necessary for survival, these systems cannot keep up.

The body has a master hormone system that is rationing out sex and stress hormones, among other intricate chemical processes. I like to imagine a large umbrella as the master hormone supervisor. Under the arch, rather than one handle, there are two. On one side, the supervisor is directing the production of sex hormones. On the other side, he's formulating cortisol or the "stress hormone." When the body is in high demand for stress hormones, it begins to shift to compensate for the high production of cortisol. Essentially, robbing Peter to pay Paul. To continue this demand, the body begins to suffer from a lack of energy directed to other necessary hormone replenishment.

Chronic stress will exaggerate symptoms, sometimes visibly and other times internally where you are not in tune with the breakdown on the inside. This is why it is important to measure. Some tests can measure your cortisol levels and patterns, but often a simple feeling of "tired but wired" or even sheer exhaustion can be a clear signal that something is wrong. Whether your cortisol is high or low, either can be a sign of distress.

Your body cannot physically do any restorative or healing work when you are in the nervous system's sympathetic or "fight or flight" mode. In other words, you are not able to help your body get the support it needs. As with any diagnosis, there is necessary healing and preserving this energy to support restoration which requires you to be in the "rest and digest" or parasympathetic mode of the ANS.

When you are pulling your body's internal fire alarm repeatedly throughout the day, you are prompting a cortisol response. When cortisol is chronically elevated, your body will no longer be able to recover to homeostasis, or a state of balance, as it naturally does.

Learning to manage stress can have powerful benefits. It can truly restore your body's systems to running efficiently and effectively.

To reduce your stress level, begin by removing as many of the stressors in your day through the various practices below. Next, for the unavoidable stressors, practice your perception and response.

Tips For Reducing Daily Life Stressors

- *Look to remove as many stressors as possible*
  Do you remember the list above outlining environmental stressors ranging from food sensitivities to bacterial infections to an overly intense exercise routine? These are the stressors you may be able to remove or at least minimize. Knowledge is the first step. Getting tested to rule out or identify infections and toxic loads can provide answers that will allow for prompt action.

- *Stop watching the news*
  Removing news exposure is a life-changer. The news puts your mind into a place where you

151

automatically imagine your tragedy. What you don't realize is your brain doesn't know the difference between a real and imagined scene. When you are formulating the story in your mind of how terrible it must be to experience what the person on the news is reporting on, your body can physically take on the chemical stress response, resulting in a dress rehearsal for something that has never happened to you nor is it likely that it ever will. It is not your job to take on the sadness of all that is wrong in the world.

- *Manage your time*

  Time-management is key to eliminating stress. Tremendous programs exist to teach time management, including daily journals that keep you focused. The more prepared and structured you are in your daily routine, the more effective you are at handling things that come at you unexpectedly.

- *Create automation in your day*

  Most people have non-negotiable items in their day that they don't even have to think about, like brushing your teeth. For some, exercise takes no second thought. For others, meditation is just a part of their life that is going to happen no matter what. Most people find time in their day to get dressed. These are automated activities.

Once you have identified the stressors you can manage, what about the ones that you can't, such as the job you hate or the lack of sleep from being a caretaker? It's important to learn to react to the unavoidable stressors in a way that serves you and the people in your life. You may not be able to eliminate these stressors but you can change your response.

Tips For Improving Your Perception And Response

- *When a stressor presents, use tools like breathing* Breathing can be done anywhere, for any duration, even several seconds, and be beneficial to the body. There are several ways to practice breathing. Breathing can be done in a car, in your office, or any place you find yourself triggered by stress. A little bit goes a long way.
- *Ask yourself, "What am I able to control?"*

Soon you will realize the situation is likely going to unfold in an unknown way. That is when you surrender your control and decide instead to remain calm because the alternative of reacting with anger or doubt will only cause you to suffer more. Staying present in a moment of anticipation will keep you from predicting an outcome and getting stuck in that dress rehearsal for trauma again.

- *What if you are waiting on health test results until the end of a week?*

That's the worst! The time has to pass. You can choose to experience it passing in a joyful, peaceful way, knowing you will jump whatever bridge that is coming your way with whatever you need to get over it. *Or* you can attempt to predict the outcome, filling your mind with all of the possibilities, good and bad, while never knowing what will happen at the end of that week. No amount of stress will make the outcome any different, but it will certainly steal every ounce of happiness you may have in each moment leading up to it.

- *Lead with compassion*

  Imagine you had the opportunity to know the story of the person in the car that just cut you off. You assume he's careless or texting or just not paying attention and was personally inconsiderate of you and your car on the road. Then you find out that man had received a call from the police explaining his son had been in an accident and he didn't know if he was going to see his son alive ever again as he raced to the hospital. You do not know the reasons for people's actions, you can only control yourself. Therefore, leading with compassion brings an inner calm versus the assumption the other person is out to get you.

- *Assume each person has a story*

  Even if it's just a rude salesperson. The person could have had a terrible morning as she is a caretaker to her sick mother and is overwhelmed with grief and stress. You may never actually learn the story of another, but if you always lead with compassion, you still win. On days when the diagnosis is getting the best of you, you would

155

hope for that same compassion. The other person's attitude is not personal.

Stress is another topic that can be in a book of its own. When you search "books on stress" on Amazon, you get seventy-five pages of results! Let's just say it is a topic of significant importance. People I see overlook the true and severe impact the stress response has on the body. Look for more on stress management in later chapters.

In conclusion, before POTS, I did not have the experience or the wisdom to understand how nutrition, stress, and sleep were contributing to my body's erosion. Nutrition and lifestyle changes are such a hugely critical aspect of healing your body from POTS. Changing your nutrition can bring about more energy, better sleep, improved digestion, beautiful skin, and cellular healing. Improved sleep may lead to better focus, hormone balance, and weight management. Minimized stress can mean improved health, a decrease in symptoms, and a balance of mind and body. There are layers to this step and it takes time and patience to learn and unlearn all of the information we think we already know.

We are a society full of information, but at the end of the day what we most seek is wisdom. In other words, we have access to answers and endless facts, but the application of this knowledge and using good judgment is what takes practice. We don't "know" something unless we are doing it.

Exercise: Monitoring Your Energy Quota

Something as simple as getting dressed can create a list of decisions that is a mile long. Do I wear a long skirt or pants? Red or blue? No, it's too hot, I think I will go with the white. Oh, no I wore that last week! All of this blah blah blah in your mind is stealing your very precious energy and taking away from your decision-making quota for the day.

You may wake up and stir in bed thinking, should I go to the gym? I could go later. No, I won't go later. Just hit *snooze!* I need more sleep. I may feel lousy about myself. I should just get up and go." Ugh! The drama we create for ourselves! If you imagine energy being sucked from a full tank throughout the day, where would your tank be by noon? Each decision we make is emptying our energy fuel tank.

Decision fatigue is a phenomenon causing paralyzing effects where our lack of energy and focus leads to poor decision making. Ever notice how late in the day, you are likely to give in to something that earlier in the day may have been more resistible? Filling more of your day with non-negotiables will allow you to be more resilient to the stressors of the day because you won't have to contemplate every single thing you do. The experience of contemplating and then beating ourselves up is a stressor in itself.

- Plan your action items. Assess your day the night before. Complete the top three priority items in your day *early*. Once they are complete, productivity will soar!

- Plan your workouts and meals. Don't go into the day with no clue when and what you will eat. Set yourself up for success by having veggies cut up, prepared protein sources, and handy clean snacks if you are forced to eat on the run.

- Plan what you will wear. Eliminate wasted energy by picking out clothes the night before.

- Plan how you will feel. Practice your gratitude and affirmations the night before or at the start of your day, always including one˙ thing that supports how you *desire* to feel, even if you aren't there yet emotionally.

CHAPTER 6

"YOU DON'T LOOK SICK" – FINDING YOUR TRIBE

"Sometimes the only answer people are looking for when they ask for help is that they won't have to face the problem alone."

– Mark Amend

When it comes to POTS, often we spend so much time faking being well that people don't even realize the struggle on the inside. It's important to lean on someone who "gets it."

For me, that was my mom. After she passed, my sister slipped into the role and took an interest in being by my side. I'll never forget the first trip to the hospital that I did solo. I was in my triage room waiting for my

IV, feeling vulnerable and alone. From behind the curtain, I saw my sister's head pop in. She had her "hospital goodie bag" she used to carry around for both Mom and Dad. It was full of entertaining things like books, an iPad, snacks, phone chargers, sweaters, socks – all the things you may need if your visit is extended for any reason.

With tears in my eyes, I felt guilty. I knew I would be okay. I knew my sister didn't have time to be hanging in a hospital with me. But, wow, did it feel so good to have her there. She reassured me there was nowhere she would rather be, and at that moment, I believed her.

When you are down and out, you have to learn to receive love and care. Dismissing someone's attempts to be there for you is insulting to the person expressing their love. You are taking away from them the wonderful feeling of giving.

You need someone who understands what you go through. They will validate you and be your biggest cheerleader. They can look at you and see the strength and courage no one else recognizes. As Cory Booker once said, "And sometimes asking for help is the most meaningful example of self-reliance."

Frequently, when you consistently exhibit strength and independence, people don't think you need any help. Some people may reject the idea of you needing anyone or anything.

I go back to a time when I could have used a hand. My dog had been sick and just been released after spending the night at the vet. The next morning, I woke to find her worse than before. I had a big work presentation that morning and could not figure out a way to juggle getting her to the vet, getting myself to my meeting, and getting her a ride home. On top of this, I was sick myself with a nasty cold and struggling to make it through the morning in the first place. I rarely ask for help with anything, so when I found myself trying to call and text my then-boyfriend and he did not answer or return my texts, I was disappointed.

I finally found my sister and she agreed to pick up Mia and bring her home for me, assuming she would be released.

My boyfriend and I were working through some things in therapy around that time. The incident with the

163

dog came up and when the therapist asked him how he felt hearing me say that I needed him and he wasn't there, his response was "Leslie is resourceful." I was confused, a little angry, and didn't know whether to take it as a compliment or as validation that I was better off taking care of things myself and not asking for help.

The point is because I always took care of things myself, he felt I would always find a way. What was the big deal that he wasn't there? I got it done.

Don't be afraid to ask for help. You don't have to be resourceful all of the time. You don't have to wear the superhero cape 24/7. It feels nice to have people be there for you. It feels even nicer for them to feel like they are doing something helpful.

Finding and building your support system is a big deal. You need more than one or two people, because, occasionally, you'll find that people you always thought would have your back may drop from your circle altogether.

An example from my history demonstrates this (perhaps you have a similar experience of your own). When I was diagnosed with POTS, I was living with a friend. She and I shared almost all of our time outside of

164

work together. We were very social, and I used to enjoy that glass (or bottle) of wine each time I got home from a stressful day. We were both single, too, so we enjoyed going out to dinner and bars and spending some afternoons enjoying lunch on the water with an umbrella drink in hand.

I was at the height of POTS when my mom was diagnosed with cancer. By that time, I had stopped drinking and was leading a very restricted lifestyle. I was fortunate to be able to spend a lot of time with Mom during her chemo treatments and taking her to doctor's appointments.

This was when the trouble started with my roommate. I will never be able to dismiss from my mind the blow-out I had with who used to be one of my best friends. My roommate declared via text, "You are depressing to be around." Our lives had gone in different directions and she was going to move out.

I was in the pits of fear for my mom, trying to keep my head above water, and reading those words was so painful. I attempted to defend myself, citing the changes since I got sick; my roommate argued that I was not sick at all.

That was the end of an otherwise beautiful friendship. It was also the beginning of me being very selective of the people with whom I would surround myself moving forward.

Incredibly, shortly after my mom passed, I met new, amazing, health-conscious people through my fitness studio. They not only looked out for me and supported me but they were also my new tribe. I always maintain my Earth Angels were handpicked by my dear Mother in Heaven.

SOCIAL SUPPORT AND PHYSICAL HEALTH

There is great research that reviewed links between social support and physical health. There is evidence that social support is essential to predicting well-being throughout all stages of life. The ability to cope with stress is highly influenced by the presence of social support.

In his paper "Relationships Between Social Support and Physical Health" (found here: http://www.personalityresearch.org/papers/clark.html),

Corey Clark of the Rochester Institute of Technology identifies six criteria for social support and their impact among adolescents, middle-aged adults, and older adults:

- Support from a lover or spouse
- Support from a group of friends or people
- Assurance of worth from others
- Reliable support
- Guidance and support from a higher figure
- Opportunity of Nurturance

Emotions and health have a significant relationship. People with positive emotions and beliefs are likely to have improved physical health. Laughter is said to have a positive impact on the reduction of stress.

While it is still early in the developments, there is a strong relationship between social and emotional support being protective of health. The associated research interestingly noted the importance of both providing support and receiving it, the various types of support, and the implications for support on various health conditions as well as the effect on mortality. [17]

Social considerations have been increasingly accepted as essential causes of health conditions. There is a need to understand the dynamics between various illnesses and types of support, but there is a positive relationship between social influences and well-being. You can read more about the social determinants of chronic disease here. [18]

While I may have lost a friend, I gained much more in the quality friendships I later attracted and nurtured. When you are going through tough times and it is hard to help people understand the types of emotions that hit you daily, it is not uncommon to affect the people who love you the most. The shame and guilt of sometimes being short and snippy with family or friends are tough on both sides, so it is important to acknowledge your loved ones and express how much you appreciate the help they give to you.

WHEN THEY DON'T HAVE YOUR BACK

Many people are not so lucky to have people in their lives on whom they can depend. They often grow up in a place with very little support and still struggle with their family relationships. It is important to understand their history and their early experiences in life, as well as their current situation, to truly help them find the comfort they need. If you *are* one of these people, overcoming the absence of help is completely doable.

When I coach clients with a lack of support, I start by reviewing their timeline. Together, we talk about their early memories and any symptoms that developed in various stages of their history. Understanding adverse childhood experiences is important not only in assessing how they will cope with POTS but also in determining how best to help them develop trust and recognize the availability of the support for which they are starving. These experiences can include but are not limited to:

- Physical, emotional, or sexual abuse
- Parental divorce
- Incarceration of a parent
- Alcohol or drug abuse
- Economic hardships
- Exposure to neighborhood violence

169

Adverse Childhood Experiences (ACE) like these are linked to multiple adverse health outcomes. A 2013 study looking at adverse childhood experiences and diagnosis of cancer found the association between ACEs and adulthood cancer may be attributable to disease progression through the association of ACEs with risk factors for other chronic diseases. In the study, ACEs are categorized into three groups: abuse, neglect, and family/household challenges. You can read that study in full here. [19]

According to the CDC-Kaiser ACE Study [20], ACEs are common. Almost two-thirds of the study participants reported at least one ACE, and more than one in five reported three or more.

The Kaiser-ACE study revealed that as the number of ACEs increased, so did the following:

- Alcoholism and alcohol abuse
- Chronic obstructive pulmonary disease
- Depression
- Death
- Health-related quality of life
- Ischemic heart disease

- Liver disease

- Poor work performance

- Financial stress

- Smoking

- Suicide attempts

This is a shortened list of potential outcomes. When I'm looking at POTS or another chronic illness in my clients, I find it is important to evaluate the ACE score to establish the type of support the individual might need. For example, a person with few quality friends, a disconnected family that lives out of town, and has a history of physical abuse is going to have different recommendations than that of a person who grew up with loads of support and a strong family unit.

The bottom line is that if you've had a difficult past, you can't afford to go it alone. You need others around you. Fortunately, when you don't have the luxury of a familial support system, there are other means to find encouragement and assistance. As Brené Brown said, "You can't get through courage without walking through vulnerability."

Finding your tribe is a critical step when dealing with POTS. You don't need people to completely understand every little thing you are feeling. And they won't, because it is not their experience. You need people who love you anyway. The people who will push you when you need to be encouraged, but know when it is enough. The people who will nurture you when you just need someone to take care of you. The people who may not be the nurse type, but have a way of doing the errands you are not thinking about when your head is in the clouds of health. Surrender your control and allow yourself to be vulnerable.

Exercise: Find Your Tribe

While the adage "it's better to give than to receive" may be correct in that giving brings joy in exclusive ways, imagine the joy it brings others to be able to be a source of giving to you rather than always on the receiving end. Finding your tribe – especially for those of us with less support around us – often begins with this simple mindset shift. After you're ready to accept love and support, try these steps to invite more people into your life.

- *Lean on the people who love you*

  These are the people you can trust and rely upon without feeling the self-imposed pressure of a payback. Expressions of gratitude and appreciation are enough to let them know you recognize their efforts and love.

- *Enlist the encouragement of people who are in a similar situation*

  There is an abundance of social media (groups in particular) exclusive to people with various chronic conditions and diagnoses. The stories of success and hope can be a relief. To realize you are not alone is powerful. However, you need to choose your groups and online tribes as carefully as you would in your *in real life* (IRL) friends.

  o *Beware* the group that takes you down the rabbit hole of negativity. Some groups can be a dumping ground for complaining and misery. This is not the type of "people" you want to seek out as they will drain your energy rather than uplift you. I often join groups of various diagnoses to help learn about what is working and not working for people. It helps me with friends who are diagnosed, and in my coaching, to understand people's pain points and fears. But even for me, it can get too harmful to engage and observe; some groups can be worse than watching the news.

- *Join a group on Facebook unrelated to POTS and illness but rather geared toward your interests and hobbies*

  Many years ago, I found a fitness group completely unrelated to any type of grief or POTS. The group drove me to be accountable for the things I desired to change in my life. It was a group that had people with like-minded interests. I learned from the other members, I expanded my mindset, and I found friends from all over the country that I have since had the opportunity to meet in person – and it was like we knew each other our whole lives!

- *Talk to people in your social or work setting*

Share your story. So many people are going through challenges and making a connection with someone through a common thread of struggle can flourish into a strong bond.

- *Work with a health coach, a life coach, or therapist*

  I always say everyone should be in some type of therapy. We all need coaches. Coaches need coaches. Experts need coaches. The people who appear to have it perfectly together all have stories. They are not effective by simply going it alone. They have moral support in all different forms. I have multiple coaches in my life, and I am grateful for each one of them.

- *Find a virtual mentor*

  I have coaches who have no idea they are my coach. I use advisers from podcasts, the speakers at conferences, watching seminars, and even following blogs.

- *Find a meetup.com group*

  Meetup.com has local groups of almost any category. If there is not one already in existence, create your own.

175

There are tons of ways to find a tribe. When I travel to events, I meet with other nutrition-driven health people, coaches, functional medicine professionals, etcetera. I always walk away feeling as if I spent quality time with *my people* and I may have never met them before that day.

Finding your support system is a tool that has been proven to benefit my clients, myself, and even provides evidence to suggest the improvement in health status. There is no reason to go through any struggle alone and I hope this chapter encourages you to appoint a squad of peace people who will support you under any circumstance. The next chapter invites you to continue to discover, create, and learn new ways to connect, heal and grow - even in the face of POTS.

CHAPTER 7

ALWAYS BE LEARNING

"The capacity to learn is a gift; the ability to learn is a skill; the willingness to learn is a choice."

- Brian Herbert

Learning is infinite. This chapter provides reminders and advice to keep you on the path of healing. Not only is learning essential in your healing, but it is also necessary for keeping POTS at bay. Albert Einstein said, "Once you stop learning, you start dying." When you stop learning, you stop growing.

There were years of my corporate career when I was just going through the motions of life. I learned only through error at my work. I wasn't reading. I was watching political nonsense on the news. I wasn't challenging myself to experience new things. It was a very robotic life. Each day looked exactly like the day before. I could easily describe my life as a soap opera. You know, the shows you watched ten years ago – and if you were to watch an episode today, the characters are the same, the drama is repetitive, and nothing is different except the babies were all-of-a-sudden adults. You could pick up right where you left off and not have missed a beat. B-O-R-I-N-G.

It wasn't until life *after* POTS that I truly began to grow. Suddenly, I sought out knowledge again. I found podcasting and discovered that I was an auditory learner. I retained tons of information from hearing it, more so than watching something or reading the same information.

Certain books from that time changed my life. One was *The Compound Effect* by Darren Hardy. Not only did I stop watching the news after reading this book, but I also began to break up routines and habits that were beginning to own me.

Sleep Smarter by Shawn Stevenson taught me all there was to know about sleep and why it was critical in my healing. I adopted the principles in the book and dramatically improved my sleep.

It wasn't just non-fiction how-to books that influenced my growth and healing during this initial learning period. Books like *The Alchemist* by Paulo Coelho and *The Four Agreements* by Don Miguel Ruiz were influential in the way I viewed the world and my experience within it. *The Soul Frequency* by my energy healing therapist, Shanna Lee, taught me about my stories and releasing beliefs that were no longer serving me.

I also read and listened to books on every type of diet, nutrition plan, and lifestyle, which heavily influenced my personalized coaching strategies. Many were scientific books that emphasized newer research disputing common, old school beliefs around sugar and why we gain weight – books like *The Obesity Code* by Dr. Jason Fung and *The Case Against Sugar* by Gary Taubes, or books about how our thoughts affect our cells, as in *The Biology of Belief* by Dr. Bruce Lipton.

I could go on and on with the books. We have access at our fingertips to more information than ever before. Find your best method of learning and run with it. Access podcasts, audiobooks, hardcopy books, masterminds, seminars, motivational speakers, positive peers, etcetera. Surround yourself with the ocean of education; sink into it.

The importance of continued learning after a POTS diagnosis became very clear to me when I wasn't getting the answers from the *experts*. The more I learned, the more I realized how much they did not know. After all, when I was diagnosed, POTS wasn't common at all. Unless they are in active pursuit of new learning themselves, the doctors are trained to derail symptoms. Therefore, why would they dig deeper for one patient?

IT'S NOT ALL FOR NOTHING

There are endless ways to improve. Learning is a lifelong process. Besides being great for your brain and your health, personal growth will help you train to be the best version of yourself. Learning will help you pay it forward. You did not go through this pain and suffering for nothing. Conquering POTS is not a senseless quest. Statistically, the majority of people overcome POTS. This process serves as a tool to help you speed up that period of suffering. It serves as a building block to allow you to help others on their path to wellness. Pair that with the learning, and now you can teach what you've not only studied but also lived through.

Like Steve Jobs said, "You can't connect the dots looking forward; you can only connect them looking backward. So you have to trust that the dots will somehow connect in your future. You have to trust in something – your gut, destiny, life, karma, whatever."

I learned that feeling sorry for myself was useless. Applying my success in healing from POTS to helping others overcome the horrible fears and hopelessness associated with these conditions helps make my experience somehow worth more. When you can potentially help someone avoid the same mistakes or give them a small tip that made a big difference for you, why would you hold back from sharing? Your experience is not futile; it's necessary.

Learning not only about POTS but about other areas of interest is motivating and helps you to grow. With POTS, I realized how stuck I'd been, not just in living, but in my health and how I wanted to feel daily.

Learning is free. Asking yourself insightful questions is empowering and opens up doors to more freedom.

Conventional medicine wants to name a disease, then blame it, and finally "treat" it with medications. This does not mean we must do the same. As with any experience in your life, find the reason why. Consider how this trial is an opportunity for you. This is your journey; it's part of who you have become. Be grateful for the relationship. Take the good with the bad. It happened *for* you, not *to* you. If it wasn't for your health challenge, you wouldn't know your strength and determination. If it wasn't for feeling awful, you wouldn't know your gratitude for feeling good.

We may not see it when we are in the middle of the mess, but somewhere inside of the experience, we grow into something better and stronger. Everything that is a struggle will build you into who you were meant to be. As Joel Osteen said, "Only God can turn a mess into a message, a test into a testimony, a trial into a triumph, a victim into a victory."

IT'S NEVER ONE THING

Our minds like a simplistic view. Very much like a computer, you input data A and get output B. But health is more complex than that. *Wellness is about various factors.* The input is copious: environmental factors, nutrients, sleep quality, stress management, supplementation, skincare, electromagnetic fields, GMO's, water purity, etcetera. And even if you have them all mastered, it does not guarantee the output you might expect.

It took a long time for most people to get to POTS, even if it came on suddenly. It isn't likely a single thing that created the problem. The body was vulnerable before the trigger set off the dominos of symptoms. Similarly, it won't be one single solution that will fix it. It's more like A + B + C + D + E *may* = positive outcome. However, even that equation isn't straightforward all the time; you may need a little more of A, less of C, moderate amounts of D, and a ton of E to get to the outcome you want. This formula takes experimentation, and that takes time. But our brains are uncomfortable with waiting – which is another reason why gratitude is so important.

I bring this up here because learning is part of keeping up the work you have done and continue to do. I certainly did not know to pay attention to these efforts early in my struggle with POTS. I learned over the years of process of elimination and investigation.

This is also why it is so important to stay ahead. We like to think things sneak up on us and we did not see them coming, but often, we are just in denial. If your car's "service now" light was illuminated, would you ignore it? When you are out of gas, do you refill your tank to the maximum or do you fill it just enough to get you through another day or two?

This distinction always fascinates me. My mom would never let her car go below half a tank before she'd fill back up. Most people I know will drive around on fumes well after the gas light has flashed before they will slow down long enough to refuel their tanks – even if they realize running out of gas will be a big waste of time and a much bigger hassle versus just pulling over and filling up now. One approach is driven by the investment of time and the other is driven by the desire for safety, of never risking being low on fuel.

When you step out of the identity of POTS and become the CEO of your health, you are never low on fuel. You don't wait for the warning lights to come about. You are ahead of schedule. You aren't interested in quick-fixes or delayed responses. You embrace being one step ahead, which, in turn, gives you the freedom to live fully. Like John F. Kennedy said, "The time to repair the roof is when the sun is shining"

In Florida, we prepare for hurricanes each year. But coming off of a beautiful winter and spring, we tend to forget all the damage we suffered in years prior. When you live in hurricane land, you don't wait around for things to fall apart before you strengthen your foundation. Being on top of things allows you to react quickly and put out a small fire before it becomes a full out scorching flame.

In essence, you can position yourself in a place of power before POTS begins to take over your life. You don't have to be married to the diagnosis for years. You may have a short courtship. Sometimes the early red flags allow you to dodge a bigger bullet or even a

185

torpedo! Executing on the critical steps in this book can speed up your healing and lead you to a place of peace and positivity faster than you can imagine.

If you're reading this book, maybe you have POTS or another diagnosis but feel great right now and have for some time. I'd argue that this is the best time to put more energy into you're your wellness – while you have the ability and time to focus on something other than your symptoms (that "check engine" or "low fuel" light.)

GET IN ON THE ACTION

Personal growth requires participation. If nothing changes, nothing will change. To continue your education and healing successfully, you must go out and pursue growth. You can't do better unless you know better, so it's critical to do the homework. One of my favorite statements to live by is "how you do anything is how you do everything."

I have been an avid Pilates student for over eighteen years. I loved it so much that I decided to get certified to teach about five years ago. Teaching a class
186

can go way beyond teaching the simple skill of an exercise. For me, it's an opportunity to preach a bigger message about commitment and intentional learning.

Today, I teach a class once a week for fun. I enjoy being on the microphone teaching up to eighteen students in a class. I continually remind them of this idea: "How you do anything is how you do everything." When they come into class, I look for enthusiasm, performance, and focus. If they walk in with poor posture, a crabby look on their face, or are not moving with the flow of the class, I bring it to their attention. If they are reluctant in their movement and lack intention with their body language, it will reflect on other aspects of their day and in their life. If you come to class half-assed and expect results, you are likely going to get more of the same and wonder why your body isn't changing. When you do things with a smile, without resistance, and put your best foot forward, it is likely the other actions in your life reflect this positive attitude and self-assurance.

This attitude is a starting place for personal growth. My instructor, friend and mentor, Ellen Latham, maintains that *Showing up is not enough. You must come to perform.* You are looking to execute on behaviors that

187

will help you achieve the separation from the diagnosis label you have been living with for too long. Divorcing your diagnosis takes effort. It is work that does not always come without struggle. Understanding this and pursuing it anyway is where the courage comes in. It's how your inner warrior comes to life.

What else can you do, then, to participate actively in your growth?

Aside from reading and learning from resources like podcasts and the internet, in-person events are incredibly useful. Attending conferences can be life-altering. Surrounding yourself with inspiring people and experts on wellness or other topics that you are passionate about changes your momentum. Being with others can lift you and shift your energy, propelling you more toward your desired result. You can meet amazing, like-minded people and hear stories of powerful recoveries. My presence at a conference influenced the writing of this book!

POTS is not your destiny if you believe in freedom from the diagnosis. Circumstances do not define who you are as a person. Hopefully, as you have read throughout this book, you've seen that I have not set aside respect and honor for POTS. When taking control of POTS, there is no disregard for reality. Rather, there is a *choice* to change your perception of reality and look at it from a different set of lenses. Add in a touch of focus on attracting what you most desire, and things may begin to shift, as you will see in the next section.

PRACTICE THE LAW OF ATTRACTION

In the early days of POTS, I was not very connected to my inner being. I was not "centered," if you will. I was not body-aware or focused on the role my thoughts played on my healing nor my erosion.

I was struggling to find a place in the book for this topic of Law of Attraction, as I believe it has so much influence on my continued healing and keeping up the ability to stay independent from letting the POTS diagnosis dictate my life, as well as any diagnoses I could face in my future. The Law of Attraction states you will attract into your life that on which you focus.

The Law of Attraction is easy to oversimplify, leaving people to dismiss it as inconsequential. It is a hard concept to grasp for people who feel like doing more results in bigger outcomes. The truth is, the Law of Attraction offers a bit of *relief* from the chase. Instead, it proposes a relaxed state of faith and working in line with a particular vibration – one that shines a light on the enormous potential for abundance in all areas of your life.

I don't mean to give the impression that hard work is not still applicable, but operating on the path of least resistance allows your efforts to flow with the least amount of controlled effort. When you resist a situation, you feel the angst of what you believe *should happen.* Often, disappointment is followed by judgment. You can't turn back time. Life is always trying to push us forward. When you feel stuck, it just that you have stopped.

Finding an easier path can help to unstop your progress. But we, as humans, are not as inclined to "allow." We have to work at this allowing thing. It's natural for us to resist, rather than let things play out. As Lao Tzu said, "Those who flow as life flows know they need no other force."

The Law of Attraction places you in the role of creation, meaning you create your reality by the things on which you choose to focus. In other words, you get back what you put out. There are more complexities than this, but for purposes of drawing better things into your world, let's keep it simple.

The teachings of Abraham-Hicks have an interesting approach to the Law of Attraction. I find it impossible to accurately describe the teachings of Abraham and I would caution that it takes attention and deep understanding to tap into the power of the enlightenments proposed by Esther Hicks, but if you can find the patience, it can truly alter your belief in how much control you truly have in creating experiences in your life. Esther Hicks acts as a conduit for the essence of Abraham as she channels the teachings from another realm. You can learn more about Esther Hicks through her writings, videos, and/or seminars.

Abraham-Hicks maintains that "The basis of your life is freedom. Your life is joy." No matter which way you receive their encouragement, there is no arguing their teachings unless you would like to dispute the benefits and desires to live a happy, joyful life.

191

The reason I bring up Abraham-Hicks is I had the opportunity to see Esther Hicks this past year at her live event. I had stumbled upon her work a couple of years ago at random on Pinterest, probably looking for a recipe. I clicked on a thirty-minute discussion that shifted my thought process so much that I shared it with everyone that would listen and I played it over and over again, finding new little nuggets of wisdom with each new presentation.

I started to follow their work and I found in times when my spirits were not fully driven from a place of love, I would find joy and peace from hearing their enlightenments. They would immediately lift me and shift me into action. If I was living or acting in fear, I was able to lead with love instead, and everything changed at that moment. My attitude changed to one of hope. I felt lighter. I believed again I would feel peace from POTS. I called into my life more love.

Call it gratitude or mindfulness, but whatever it was, it was quick, powerful, and effective in maintaining the disengagement and freedom from POTS symptoms. Amazingly, the message was consistent with the expressions of my energy healing therapist, who always

192

encouraged me to act from a place in my heart rather than apprehension.

Thanks to Abraham-Hicks, I began to pay attention to my focus and where my mind liked to hang out. I observed my thoughts and feelings like never before. I had always described myself as one of those people who knew what I didn't want but had no idea what I *did* crave. After realizing that as humans, we are meant to learn through all of life's contrast, I was learning to take what I didn't want and reframe quite the opposite to become very clear on the feeling I most hungered for. Until I was ready and able to recognize how I wished to feel, I had remained in the clarity of its opposite – that which I had *no* desire to feel. For example, in looking for a partner, you may know for certain you *do not* wish to meet an unreliable person. Rather than focusing on the lack of reliability, the focus would be on the feeling of significance and certainty. The feeling that you are supported and have dependable people in your life is where your focus is best held.

Once I realized how I'd been blocking myself – by focusing on the negative side of clarity – that's when I began to get more of what I most needed. I paid attention to how I *felt*. I reiterated in my journaling and gratitude all of the pleasurable feelings such as healthful, energetic, joy, peace, love, clarity, wonder, laughter, comfortable, calm, abundant, etcetera. Shortly after consistently focusing on these delightful feelings, more circumstances appeared in my life that generated more of them.

The Law of Attraction may not be perceivable, but if you pay attention, you will see it in action. A great example was one day when I was avoiding a particular person – so much so that I had gone out of my way to predict her whereabouts to not run into her. I had asked other people if she was around. I had even looked at an event online that I suspected she may be attending out of town. When I had concluded I was probably in the clear, I set out to walk my dogs that late Saturday afternoon and *bam* – the first person I saw was the very person I had been evading all day.

The more you think about and direct your attention to something, the more you attract that very thing – whether it is serving you or not. But you can use this to your advantage in planning what you want to bring into your life. I have used this methodology in the

194

development of my vision boards. Similar to my recordings of the ideal future and the visual details of my dreams coming to life, these boards are the physical images and manifestations of my audacious goals. I started these ten years ago. Today, I have many years of vision boards in which I created the things I most wanted to see in my world.

Each year, I create my new board with my sister and some friends (see the end of the chapter for exercise on creating your very own vision board). I look back at the boards from the years past as I develop my new board. I am still astonished by how many details of the boards became a reality. And anything that had not yet come to pass was simply transferred onto my new board because I still invested hope and patience into the dream's birth.

DON'T JUST TAKE MY WORD FOR IT

I know this might all sound a bit magical and woo-woo. But don't knock it until you try it. Whether you believe it or oppose it, it is not mythical. It is science.

Just like gravity is an unchanging law of the universe, so is the Law of Attraction. Believe it or not, it is a straight-up universal principle. If you choose to understand it and practice, you may see things start to fall into place and the continuity of your healing and freedom from POTS symptoms becomes more and more certain.

There are 7 Laws of Attraction:

1. Unwavering desire
2. Conceptualization and imagination
3. Affirmation
4. Focus with confidence
5. Profound belief
6. Gratitude
7. Manifestation

You'll notice we have already covered many of these concepts as part of the critical steps to healing from diagnosis, POTS in particular.

You may start by honestly becoming clear on what you truly want. Many people simply just do not know, as I didn't. If they do have an idea, they are not very clear on the details of it.

For instance, the question I ask people about what an ideal day is when they are feeling their best. The more detail they can provide, the more specific they are, the better the clarity and potential for the manifestation. The people who have very little idea about what that might look like because they are very stuck in the mud of POTS may have a harder time getting to where they want to be because they just are not sure. As Esther Hicks said, "Rather than being so ready to jump into action to get the things that you want, we say think them into being; see them, visualize them, and expect them – and they will be."

What is cool is when you picture where you stand in your life today, we tend to have a vision of getting from point A to point B in our lives. However, we don't get there from here. Instead, if we prepare here at point A, where we are, and learn to be happy in our current reality, then *there (point B)* comes over *here.* Think about this. You are not moving toward a feeling. You have the power to feel the feeling through your thoughts, which leads to more of these powerful thoughts that draw to you more of the feeling you desire the most. When you calmly practice both gratitude for where you are, and a vision for where you want to be, that's when the traveling happens. Envisioning where you want to be helps to draw that new truth unto you.

Our conditions are only unchangeable because we think they are. But they're not. Imagine painting a picture. When you mess up, you can always paint over the mistake and begin on a fresh canvas. In life, we can also create fresh beginnings. Yesterday is gone. Start working off of a clean canvas. You have the opportunity and the choice to do this at any given moment. It takes practice and focus and using the tools consistently as presented in this book.

It's easy to make things on the surface look right. Especially in the state of chronic disease, we may look one way but feel a very different way on the inside. If we walked around with our insides on the outside, we would be way too vulnerable. But what if we created our inside to be bright and peaceful in spite of our body's disagreement? What if we focus on healing in the depths of our soul, then let the exterior just happen? The light on the inside can beam right through beyond the surface. When you do the inside work, you feel the world around you shift. This is an example of the Law of Attraction as it relates to POTS.

Everything is created twice. You think it before you create it. Something has to be a thought before it emerges into reality. Just like we talked about thoughts becoming beliefs.

As human beings, we have to be aware of what we are thinking because what we feed grows. We must also be aware of our tendency to shuffle around in chaos to match up with the ever so common chaotic lifestyle of today's world. If your mind carries a heavy thought pattern, you will experience more of the same. Heavy can mean the weight of the world. Thoughts of dread or stressful situations or even the horrific happenings in the world over which we have no control overwhelm us. The thought processes will perpetuate themselves so rather turn around that heavyweight and focus on things that feel light. Use that very same mindful pattern to serve your body and experience. Esther Hicks has said that "Life is always in motion, so you cannot be "stuck.'"

EXPERIENCE IS A GIFT

Becoming aware of the language you use with others as well as with yourself is an essential step in creating that ideal life you have now envisioned. Talking to others about how bad you feel or gossiping about others will continue to bring more ill will to light. Going out of your way to not discuss how badly you may feel at that moment or what a terrible week it has been or how that person is acting annoyingly will help to create a sort of happy bubble that cannot be penetrated by undesirable thoughts and discussions.

At the beginning of my journey, it was hard for me to see why POTS happened "for me" and not "to me," especially when I was in the heart of the despair that came with POTS and the uncertainty of my health consequence. I used to feel so much helplessness. I felt so defeated.

But the more you concentrate on the problem, the more you are using your imagination to create something you don't want. The more I felt sorry for myself and wondered, "Why me?", the more discouraged I would feel. It wasn't until I decided to appreciate the things that were changing for the positive in my life and give voice to them verbally that I began to see more and more positive around me. The things that were working expanded. My complaints became weaker. Of course, I was doing the work in my mindset, health, and lifestyle, but this tool – speaking of the good things – proposed on an entire new elevated level of possibility and growth.

Today, I can look back and see the benefit the experience of being diagnosed has brought to my life. POTS led me to become so much more than I had been permitting myself to be. The diagnosis drove me to strive for more after I was able to release it as my sole identity.

You see, I would never insinuate any diagnosis or disease would possibly be easy to overcome. It's the hardest thing I have ever done, outside of surviving the pain of losing my parents. But the loss of my parents also fuels my fire to become a better version of myself.

Exercise: Create the Vision

A vision board, also called a dream board, is a visualization tool. It is a reminder of life goals and things you dream about for your future. Your design is to provide a source of inspiration. As we have talked about with the Law of Attraction, what you focus on expands, so the idea is the energy you shift towards your passions and desires will draw them towards you. This exercise is good for both starting and for starting over, but also for maintaining during the tough times when you lose sight of what you want.

I am a true testament to this exercise. I did my first vision board with some friends years ago as part of a women's group activity. I had none of my materials in hand. I just showed up. I was still working in corporate and had not imagined my life any further ahead of getting through the next day, not because I was present, but because I was stressed all of the time.

When I arrived, we sat around a table and cut out pictures and quotes from magazines – items that represented our dreams for the future. Then we pasted them onto small boards. I felt like I had very few things on my board, but I felt accomplished after participating in what I saw as a fun, social exercise. At the end of the evening, I took the board home and propped it behind my nightstand in the bedroom.

A couple of years later, I had left corporate and was working from home. I noticed the board peeking out from behind the nightstand. When I pulled it out, I was surprised at what I saw. All of the little cut-outs, sayings, and pictures were a reality in my current world. My visions had come true.

I did my next vision board with my sister and some friends and saw similar results. Over time, these little dream board parties became an annual ritual. Each year, I reflect on the prior year and realize the blessings that have come to life. I also appreciate my role in the creation of these blessings, as they were all things I had once only imagined or dreamed about.

These boards aren't magic. But the process of building one helps you to get clear on what you desire most. When you are clear on your intentions, the consistent action that follows is what takes you to the level of actualization. Even if it sounds too airy-fairy for you, what do you have to lose?

My boards have become much more elaborate and detailed these days. I use a lot of color, sparkle, glitter, stickers, and other fun supplies. The goal is to keep it positive and to express what brings you joy.

Ideally, the vision is from your perspective or looking through your own eyes. For example, if you want to be a speaker, you might use a photo of an audience you would see as you are standing on stage versus a photo from the lens of someone *in* an audience, viewing the speaker on stage. This is just one tip, but there are no real "rules" that I follow. The only "rule" is to let yourself dream.

How to Create Your Vision Board

1. *Gather up some supplies*

   Poster board (I use full-sized), magazines of interest, personal photos, quotes, stickers, glue sticks, markers, colorful paper, scissors, etcetera. You can get some of these things from a craft store specifically designed for these types of projects.

2. *Find a large area to set up shop*

   Make sure you have enough space for all of your goodies to spread out. Create an atmosphere of joy. You may play music or share stories with friends, or burn candles, or even sit in silence.

3. *Begin with intention by asking yourself some thoughtful questions*

- What is it that you want?
- What words describe how you wish to feel?
- What do you value most?

4. *Find images and words that match up to your intentions*

   You can always create your own if you cannot find the exact language that resonates with your creation. Select things that bring out peace and feelings of well-being. Avoid images of comparison.

5. *Assemble your board*

   You may paste as you go or line things up and put it all together at one time. Add your finishing touches and assess how it feels to look at your creation.

6. *Place your board somewhere that you can see it*

   Look at your board frequently and connect with the desires that made you choose the images you selected.

7. *Remember your "why."*

   The bigger reason for your dreams is your why. Why do you desire these changes? What feelings will you gain by these dreams coming to life?

205

What is the bigger reason for making these dreams coming true?

A vision board is a fun exercise. If you take it for what it is and keep your heart light and faithful, you might just find yourself taking action steps that support the very dreams you are wishing to come true.

Staying divorced from a diagnosis requires continued effort, education, loyalty to the critical steps, and thoughtful, committed practices. Your vision board is simply another way to bring your body and mind back to a state of harmony. As Helen Keller said, "The only thing worse than being blind is having sight, but no vision."

And it's fun. Fun is healthy. So, there's that.

This chapter has many deep concepts that take time to adopt. Going through the motions of the questions and building on your dreams takes courage and an open mind. Take your time. Enjoy the process. In the meantime, the next chapter will truly help you to build on these efforts.

CHAPTER 8

NAIL TRUE RESILIENCE

"We must embrace pain and burn it as fuel for our journey."

– Kenji Miyazawa

Resilience is the capacity to recover quickly from difficulties or to bounce back. Resilience is the ability of your body to rapidly return to normal, both physically and emotionally, after a stressful event. However, some people are naturally more resilient to stress than others. People with the most natural resilience tend to have a higher tolerance for stress. That is not always a good thing. When your mind says "I got this" all of the time, you begin to ignore that your body still has a physiological response to perceived stress. Let me explain.

In my curiosity about all things health, I participated in my first biofeedback session on a trip to Canyon Ranch in Tucson, Arizona. In biofeedback therapy, you are connected to electrical sensors that help you to receive information about your body. These instruments are used to measure various aspects of your physiological responses, including brainwaves, heart rate changes, sweat response, body temperature, respiratory rate, or pain perception, among others. Biofeedback can help you to gain control over normally involuntary functions and can be effective to treat physical and mental health issues, especially those driven by stress.

At the start of my session, I was asked to imagine the most stressful time in my life. I took myself back to the last moments of my mom's life. I recalled the way she was breathing, the sound of the oxygen machine, the grief that sat heavy on my chest, my inability to breathe imagining her no longer being physically in my life daily. I imagined my sister, my dad, and me holding her hands and saying our goodbyes, giving her permission to

208

let go and reassuring her we would all be okay. I could feel the tears that flooded me when she took her last breath. Even just writing this, I know in my mind, I can handle the memory, but my body is developing a lump in my throat, my muscles feel tense, and my heart is stirring.

Well, that is precisely what the sensors reflected. My heart rate changed, my sweat response kicked in, my brain waves shifted, and my body temperature adjusted.

Next, my therapist guided me to a more neutral place. Everyday activities. At that time, my dad had been experiencing a lot of physical challenges since my mom passed, so daily we were faced with some type of chaos. I recalled finding my dad on his front yard walkway, lying in the grass. When I got there, his dog Spirit stood over him in the hot Florida summer sun while he was bleeding from his face and vomiting. I looked back on the multiple ambulance rides and the constant wondering if this was going to be the day and if this was how it would end.

Interestingly, the therapist said to me, based on my body responses, he could see my thoughts had shown an initial peak response. However, whatever it was that I

209

was thinking about, he reported, my body had gotten used to. It was wild how he could see the way I had an initial stress response, but then it became stable in its elevation. My dad's health issues had become my "norm."

Once I got back down to my baseline, my therapist asked me to imagine a peaceful scene. Something that brings me calm and relaxation. I went right to horses. I envisioned riding down a beautiful road, the trees with beautiful leaves creating an arch across the top as if to shape a tunnel. I could hear the horse's hooves clip-clopping on the roadway. It was breezy and cool. I could hear the birds singing. My dogs ran along beside us. I was holding the loop in the reins at the very tip because my horse was just as relaxed and enjoying the walk as I was.

My stress responses led to an initial increase in heart rate and body temperature. Not surprisingly, while thinking about riding, my measurements went in just the opposite direction. My body responded with relaxation, a slowed heart rate, a stable body temperature, steady brain waves, and no sweat response.

I was fascinated. In one moment, with one thought, I could take my body to a place of pain and anxiety. In another moment, with one thought, I could bring my body to a place of harmony and tranquility. Biofeedback therapy had shown me evidence that the power of thoughts can completely impact your physical body and health.

I use this example with many clients to show them the effects of stress are powerful, even if they think they "got it." It also serves to demonstrate how calm, positive thoughts can be just as effective in shifting their body's responses. I see women who are rock stars at the office and champions at home, and similarly, they are trying to power through a diagnosis. I love their ability to tap into that inner strength that a person only realizes she has when she is faced with experiences she could never imagine surviving. I admire the intense determination people have for not letting a diagnosis get the best of them. This is critical to not allowing it to take over your identity.

However, I also reassure them it is okay to embrace the disheartening moments. It's okay to admit the situation sucks. Simply pretending nothing bothers us is not going to move the needle on healing.

The concept of "fake it til you make it" is powerful. And effective. It describes a person who can be very compartmental, meaning she is able to stuff away an emotion into a tiny box and put it away for the moment. Perhaps even for long periods of time. While this is critical in the process of imagining yourself well and not letting POTS define who you are, I believe *true* resilience cannot be attained without embracing the inner drama queen. When we constantly fake it and "power through" without ever allowing a moment of being human, we avoid our real emotions in real-time.

During my time with POTS and the trauma of losing my parents, I was very compartmental. I could stuff away any pain or frustration I had at any given moment. I thought, "Is there ever a good time to cry?" I couldn't cry on my way to work because it would ruin my make-up. I didn't want to cry when I was at home because I would get a headache. I couldn't cry in front of people because I didn't want people to feel sorry for me or worry. Instead, I delayed the emotion by ignoring the instinct to feel in the moment when my body and mind needed a release.

But eventually, all of these instincts to *feel* will ultimately express themselves, often in your body and health. They find their way to make it to the surface somehow. Sometimes, it is in your mental health, and often in your physical health.

When I started to get in shape after POTS, I had become an avid runner. When I felt scared for Mom, I ran. When I was stressed from Dad, I ran. When I needed a good cry, I ran. When I felt happy, I ran. I ran every single day. Not far, but enough to shake out some tears and let my body feel that "flight" response. Enough to pump chemicals to my brain to help me avoid the feelings of grief and sadness.

I ran until I hurt myself. I didn't call it my *mom hip* for nothing. I manifested so much pain and unexpressed discomfort that my body finally gave me the big *kiss-off*. Between my busted hip and hamstring and subsequent gut issues, my emotions popped out in much bigger ways than if I had just had my meltdowns as they came my way.

The more naturally resilient we are, the more often we need to check in with our bodies and minds. Emotions come in waves. To be *truly* resilient, sometimes you have to schedule a time to *fall apart.* Why? Because when you numb sadness, you also numb happiness and joy. To experience the magical feelings of pure joy, you have to know the feelings of sadness and pain.

This is probably one of the most important steps in this process. No one likes being uncomfortable, but you cannot truly recover from anything without experiencing the trauma. Learning to sit in the ugly is true resilience. The key is not to stay down there for too long.

Allowing yourself to feel pain or anger and to sit in it for a *short time* is healing. Science shows that cortisol – the body's stress hormone – is released in your brain each time you are triggered by a stressful situation. This dose of cortisol allows for added focus and chemical reactions to occur that trigger your body to react quickly to a life-threatening situation. Cortisol is ok in small doses, but our bodies were not designed to handle chronic stress daily. Unfortunately, in today's

214

world, that's the norm. Stress has been named by the World Health Organization as the Health Epidemic of the 21st Century.

So, how can we manage all this stress – both the everyday variety and the kind generated by health challenges?

Dr. Jill Bolte Taylor, a neuroanatomist (brain scientist) who dedicated her career to research into severe mental illnesses, defined the concept of "The 90-Second Rule" (her Ted Talk "My Stroke of Insight" is a remarkable watch). She says:

"When a person has a reaction to something in their environment, there's a 90-second chemical process that happens in the body; after that, any remaining emotional response is just the person choosing to stay in that emotional loop.

"Something happens in the external world, and chemicals are flushed through your body which puts it on full alert. For those chemicals to totally flush out of the body, it takes less than 90 seconds. This means that for 90 seconds you can watch the process happening, you can feel it happening, and then you can watch it go away.

"After that, if you continue to feel fear, anger, and so on, you need to look at the thoughts that you're thinking that are re-stimulating the circuitry that is resulting in you having this physiological reaction, over and over again." [21]

Tolerating an uncomfortable feeling for ninety seconds beats a lifetime of avoiding that very pain. I recall times of literally crumbling to the floor of my kitchen sobbing uncontrollably. Like something you would see in a movie. It was surreal – but so incredibly necessary. I also remember after a short time which felt like forever, I felt lighter. I *came back to my body*. I could then logically say to myself, "Where do I need to put my energy now?"

People go through so much pain trying to avoid pain. Allowing that energy to flow out of you is freeing. Dislodging those pockets of stored emotion opens up space for a new light. There is only so much real estate in your body for storage. If you plan on putting more into the unit, you have to clear out what is there first.

During my years in pharmacy, I had some amazing peers and bosses. At the peak of POTS, I was going through an unusual transition in my work setting.

216

I was blessed to have a boss who was extremely understanding and treated his team like family. We were like his kids and he had to have the humor to deal with the enormously diverse personalities of the team. His humor gave me a phrase I still use to cope today. When I would be having a rough day, he would always tell me to, *"Embrace the suck."* It turns out this is a military reference; it means *to consciously accept or appreciate something extremely unpleasant but unavoidable.* This phrase became a mantra and got me through heaps of crappy times. By embracing our lives completely, we can overcome even the things that suck.

What we have learned are ways to express true resilience. It is a skill you can practice and improve, and mastering it makes the POTS healing process more effective.

Exercise: Ways to Practice True Resilience

1. *Notice how you feel and why*

   Are you feeling sad? Why do you think that feeling is coming up right now? Show yourself a little understanding. Remind yourself you can do things to ease a sad mood and feel happier. These can be things like throwing yourself into the activities that bring you the most joy. Spend time with a good friend. Call a relative who would enjoy the surprise chat.

2. *Practice gratitude*

When you are in the middle of something sad, feel it; allow emotions to flow. Find gratitude in your body's attempt to release that stuck energy. Think positive and focus on just a few things about yourself and your situation. There is always something good – look for it. At times during a POTS flare-up, rather than resisting falling into the trap of the symptoms, I would honor the moment and simply rest. I am grateful when my body talks to me explicitly and I can listen.

3. *Stick with the truth*

Keep it simple. If you are having a bad day and just need a small pity party, cool. Make sure the invite is restricted to whatever time it takes to ride that wave. If you find the party is getting out of hand, remind yourself of the truth versus your thoughts and stories around the truth (these are all of those colorful judgments we tend to make to enhance an already elaborate story we have created in our minds). For example, I was diagnosed with POTS. That was the truth. My story was all about how debilitating my life was. My focus was on all of the crappy things that came with having POTS. I told myself I was limited. I thought about all of the things I thought I could not do. I felt self-conscious because I told myself people were judging me. All of these things were extensions of the truth of POTS. I did not need to go beyond and complicate it further. At the end of the day, the fact was there were plenty of opportunities to live my life with enthusiasm. It was up to me to inject the extraordinary in each day.

4. *Bounce back*

    How do you know when you've been down too long? When you physically don't feel like you can get back up without a helping hand. Feelings follow action. Sometimes you just have to go through the motions of standing back up, dusting yourself off, and marching proudly forward. Once you begin your march, your mind will follow. The brain grooves as your body moves. Otherwise, enlisting the help of a friend or your *person* may be just what the doctor ordered. No pun intended!

5. *Fake it 'til you make it is a real thing*

Research supports the benefits and effectiveness of acting "as if" – the idea being that if you behave like the person you want to become, you will become like this in reality. I don't mean you should be inauthentic. Acting "as if" simply means changing your behavior first and then trusting your feelings will follow. Example: did you know flashing a smile will stimulate your brain and facial muscles? You will automatically feel better. If you have a hard time smiling to yourself, place a pencil between your top and bottom teeth. Your lips are forced to be held up in a smile position. If you open your lips, the smile grows wider. Hold the pencil there for several minutes or until you feel yourself begin to lighten up…if you don't crack up at how silly you feel with a pencil in your mouth first!

6. *Just* breathe!

   Taking a deep breath with a longer exhale can shift your vagus nerve, allowing your body to shift into the parasympathetic nervous system. This is a beautiful thing to practice in the morning as it immediately calms the "rest and digest" part of the nervous system, allowing you to begin the morning fresh and in a relaxed state.

7. *Practice the 90-Second Rule*

   Most of us naturally distract ourselves before we can pause. Rather than denying a feeling as it starts to surface, acknowledge it. This practice allows you to express whatever needs an expression for ninety seconds. Do a quick journal entry. Have a meltdown. Get angry and punch a pillow. Do whatever it is that helps to relieve the feeling.

   When you're finished, it's important to decide what's next. Redirecting your brain to something productive or towards a desired feeling or thought allows you to move forward and shift to a place of calm and peace. Changing back to a "fake it until you make it" technique can also work here. You can also move into a meditative technique or consider taking two minutes to tap into your senses.

If nothing else, remember Derek Sivers's words: "Even when everything is going terribly and I have no reason to be confident, I just decide to be."

MEDITATION, MINDFULNESS, AND BREATHING

Jon Kabat-Zinn said, "Mindfulness is about being fully awake in our lives. It is about perceiving the exquisite vividness of each moment. We also gain immediate access to our powerful inner resources for insight, transformation, and healing."

Healing from a chronic syndrome or disease is not about looking away from the condition. Distraction does not address the energy it took to bring about the disease. Meditation, mindfulness, and breathing bring you to a place of conscious awareness to process and be at peace, in spite of circumstances. The power of these practices goes a long way. Small efforts add up to big benefits that can have a huge effect on your healing journey.

Mindfulness is often used interchangeably with meditation. Breathing is often mentioned with these to make up a trio of effective calming techniques. So, what's the difference?

Meditation is an umbrella term that envelops acknowledgment of thoughts and eventually deliberate consciousness. Mindfulness is a form of meditation. It is the act of focusing on being in the present.

Mindfulness can be enhanced by meditation, while meditation may expand mindfulness. There are various ways to practice both mindfulness and meditation, as well as simple breathing. They complement each other.

For me, mindfulness is being aware of the things happening on the inside and the outside. Paying attention to thoughts, emotions, feelings, and behaviors, and essentially taking yourself off of autopilot. Mindfulness can also mean tapping into all five of your senses. Noticing the smell of flowers, observing the beauty of a full moon, feeling the touch of silk, reveling in the sound of birds singing or savoring the taste of a heavenly recipe. Bringing your concentration to the present moment without judgment.

As for breathing, it's often taken for granted. Most of us do not use our full lung capacity to breathe as our lungs have more competency than we require to accomplish an everyday function. On average, a person with a healthy set of lungs only uses about seventy percent of the lung's total scope even doing intense exercise. According to vocabulary.com, "Breathing is the bodily process of inhalation and exhalation; the process of taking in oxygen from inhaled air and releasing carbon dioxide by exhalation." Because we do this without having to think about it, often we don't even notice it. Yet, we *should* be intentional breathers. Being conscious of our breathing efforts brings about strong, effective healing benefits by saturating the cells with oxygen.

Meditation, mindfulness, and breathing have powerful benefits that can remarkably impact your body. But many of us race through life without incorporating these simple, completely free, wellness techniques into our lives.

Before POTS, I knew nothing of these practices. I was completely controlled by the activities in my busy day. I was a slave to the next e-mail or the biggest "emergency." Back then, the closest I came to being mindful were my morning horse rides. I was in nature, sunshine, and had my full attention on the horse and the harmony of the movement.

When I began to learn about meditation and mindfulness, I started to introduce these practices into my routine by walking around my building several times a day at work, listening to the app Headspace. Sometimes, I would sit under a tree and spend ten minutes listening to the voice of a British guy walk me through embracing distractions and disruptive thoughts.

Little as it seemed, it was making a dent in my overactive sympathetic nervous system. I know this because I began to react to stressors, particularly at work, with more calm.

Other behaviors changed too. Before attempting mindfulness, I would listen to the early morning shows on TV in the background while I got ready for work. I would wrap up the evening with episodes of Nancy

Grace, completely enmeshed in the details of unsolved murders.

After becoming more mindful, I quit watching the news and crime shows cold turkey. The ability to begin each day without the negativity of the world helped to start me off with a clean slate. Releasing these mindless morning and evening habits was most beneficial to the pattern of my day, particularly my sleep. Going to bed with a clear mind stopped my constant dreams and nightmares, which in the past often featured the crimes I would watch right up until bedtime. My mornings and evenings were now free for more productive health building habits such as journaling and morning meditation.

FINDING YOUR MEDITATION "SOUL MATE"

Meditation is something I immediately recommend to a client, but I also recognize it is not an easy thing for people to adopt. There are so many misconceptions around meditation, such as you have to "quiet your thoughts" or that it must be practiced in a particular way to be effective or have any impact. People also struggle to wrap their heads around the possibility of meditation relieving stress in their life when they "don't have time" to practice it, to begin with. The practice is filled with judgment and reports that "I am not good at it" or "it doesn't work for me." Once I demonstrate how stress management (or lack thereof) plays a role in their physical health, they open their minds to the concept, but it still takes convincing and consistent repetitive implementation.

I believe people need to find their "soul mate" practice when it comes to exercise and meditation. You may have to try various fitness classes to find something you enjoy or can adopt as a routine. It is much harder to create a habit around something you can't stand doing than it is to do something you appreciate. But how do you do this? How do you find your meditation and mindfulness perfect fit?

I found my meditation soul mate on a women's retreat in Arizona. I met with a spiritual therapist to embark on a guided meditation described as "The Soul Journey." It was life-altering.

My soul journey began in a quiet room. I was lying down, covered with a blanket, and had a soft mask over my eyes. The therapist began by taking me through some breathing before she walked me within a visual guided meditation that felt as if I had been hypnotized but I was fully aware of my surroundings. This included the sound of drums. I wondered if it was her beating them or if it was some sort of sound therapy she was playing during our session.

Soon, my body became relaxed and my eyes saw blankets of bright purple light, which I immediately connected as the presence of my mother's soul and other spirit guides. It was so incredibly powerful, I could physically feel what I imagined to be her spirit. Dr. Ludwig took me through various scenes and as I ascended into a place that could only be thought up from the depths of an altered state, I felt a weight of pain release from my body and mind. I left the session hysterically crying – the flood of emotion was overpowering. I called my sister and sobbed as I told her of the healing I felt in every cell of my body and the release of sadness that was now flowing outside of me rather than inward.

228

It may sound woo-woo, and, quite frankly, I am okay if it was. The peace I experienced from this hour-long scene from my mind's creation was greater than years of talk therapy. Guided meditation would become my soul mate type of meditation.

From that point on, I used guided meditation through podcasts and YouTube and found I became consistent in my practice. While it is still my preference, I learned I have the capacity now to spend time in a place of silence and presence I would have never accomplished without the preparation of having someone there to keep my focus on a story. You can learn about resources for guided and independent meditation in the exercises at the end of this chapter.

I am captivated by the very different methods and impact described by the different people as meditation and mindfulness have such an exclusive, personalized effect. However, the distinct meaning the practice brings to the individual does not lessen the power. As Peter Waite said, "Mindfulness is a set of skills for healing, intuition, insight, calmness, focus, resilience and hope that you can develop to counter the stresses that chronic illness brings."

BENEFITS OF BREATHING

Though each person may practice meditation and mindfulness in their way, what all three methods have in common is attention to breath.

Breathing can cultivate mindfulness. Mindfulness, in turn, can bring about more attentive breathing. This is the reason many meditations begin by shifting your focus to your breathing and changing the tempo of the breath. You may practice elongating the exhale, which is one of the simplest, most compelling beneficial types of breathing.

I like to compare chest breathing and belly breathing. Belly breathing can often elicit an immediate relaxed response, as evidenced by the loosening of the abdomen muscles. Belly breathing is more of an east and west expansion versus chest breathing, which feels more like you are growing taller with the inhale and sinking with the exhale. East and west breathing with belly breath is more like the body expanding wide rather than tall. The midsection blows up like a Buddha-belly, distending on each side of the belly with the inhale and

230

deflating back to narrow with the exhale blowing all of the air out of the belly button.

Breathing in this way can stimulate the vagus nerve, which activates the parasympathetic nervous system. Also referred to as "diaphragmatic breathing," slowly breathing through the tummy can initiate a reduction in stress and anxiety. The vagus nerve is one of the cranial nerves that connect the body to the brain. It interchanges with the parasympathetic or "rest and digest" part of the nervous system and influences control of the heart, lungs, and digestive tract.

Deep breathing also supplies more oxygen to the brain and has a calming effect. You can utilize deep breathing any time during the day for a health benefit or calm yourself in a time of stress.

Some other health benefits of breathing include:

- *Improving the respiratory system*
  Oxygen is the most essential natural resource required by our body to survive. Deep breathing helps to release the diaphragm and primary breathing muscles, allowing the lungs to expand.
- *Calming the nervous system*
- *Improving the digestive system*

Waking up and immediately taking in several deep breaths with an elongation on the exhale can relax the bowels and make for a smooth start to the day as your body is preparing for elimination in the morning as part of our regular rhythm. [22]

- *Boosting anti-aging cellular activity*

Breathing consciously and fully does amazing things for the body. See the action steps at the end of the chapter for some wonderfully simple techniques you can use anywhere for any amount of time. A little bit goes a long way...

BENEFITS OF MINDFULNESS

Mindfulness may be used interchangeably with awareness. It is, after all, the simple act of noticing things. Have you ever made an effort to pay full attention in a situation you could have navigated with your eyes closed? I used to run with my dogs along the same path daily. I wore a headset and typically had on my blinders, only paying attention to not tripping on the paved path or jamming to my music. One day, my headset died, and in the silence, I started to listen to the sounds around me and look around. I found myself stopping and taking close up pictures of the most colorful flowers. I had not ever looked at the hedges along the path or seen so much color on any of my runs. I hadn't noticed the ripples in the water along the path or the ducks that were floating around. Now, anytime I go down that old path, I am aware of the beauty around me.

It's a completely different experience to concentrate and be fully mindful of every little thing around you. And mindfulness comes with other perks. According to the American Psychological Association, mindfulness reduces stress. The use of mindfulness-based stress reduction therapy (MBSR) has been associated with the reduction of anxiety. [23]

MBSR, a type of mindfulness meditation, was developed in the late 1970s by Jon Kabat-Zinn as a complement to medical treatment. When it comes to chronic illness, MBSR has shown to help with cancer, chronic pain, stress, anxiety, depression, fibromyalgia, and even disordered eating and Type 2 diabetes. Mindfulness can produce progress in physical and psychological symptoms and create positive changes in other aspects of well-being by:

233

- Improving mental health
- Improving life satisfaction and connectedness
- Enhancing the ability to deal with illness
- Aiding in recovery of chronic illness
- Improving academic success
- Boosting resilience
- Reducing work-related stress
- Stimulating higher brain functioning
- Increasing immune function

Given the extraordinary benefits, why wouldn't you try it?

BENEFITS AND MYTHS OF MEDITATION

As Sakyong Mipham says, "The body benefits from movement and the mind benefits from stillness." We need motion to detox and make our bodies run efficiently. On the other hand, we must be still in our mind and spirit to hear the priceless answers to life's purpose.

How do we find serenity in physical movement with mental stillness? We take the time to take pleasure in both.

You've seen the lists of benefits you can enjoy from incorporating deep breathing and simple awareness into your daily routines. Sitting in meditation offers many of the same benefits, plus some additional ones. Meditation and mindfulness can offset some of these stressful encounters in our day. They can also change your health and your brain. A small amount of time dedicated to these intentional practices can result in a large impact.

Many researchers are looking at the health benefits of meditation, along with studies that are looking deeper into how meditation works and how it affects the brain. Several potential benefits of regular meditation include the following (please note that these are all possible but not guaranteed):

- Improvements in symptoms of anxiety
- Lower blood pressure
- Improvements in quality of life by relieving stress, anxiety, fatigue, and improving sleep and general mood

235

- Improvements in pain

- Reduction in symptoms of IBS (Irritable Bowel Syndrome) and flare-ups

Meditation is not a new concept. The history goes back centuries. However, a newer report [24] shows it is becoming more and more popular, with findings that adults in the U.S. have increased the use of meditation from 4.1 percent to 14.2 percent between 2012 and 2017.

I'm happy that meditation is catching on with more people. We all can benefit. Unfortunately, many of us who need these benefits don't even try (or try and quit) because of unfortunate misconceptions.

Meditation is associated with so many myths that hold us back from dedicating our time to make it a habit. Perhaps the most common is "I don't have time." People think meditation is time-consuming or a waste of time. But the truth is, meditation helps to improve focus and reduce stress, which sets you up for more productivity and better time management.

Some argue that meditation doesn't work or they aren't able to do it right. I'd argue that the only wrong way is to not try at all. There is no right or wrong. Ideally, there is no judgment in any direction.

236

But the silliest myth I hear (perhaps one I always believed myself) is that in meditation, you are supposed to be able to stop your thoughts. That's simply not true. Meditation is about tuning in, not tuning out. You might even pay attention to some of these fleeting thoughts as part of a practice.

The best analogy I've heard comes from a wonderful expert in the area of meditation, Emily Fletcher, founder of ZIVA Meditation and author of *Stress Less, Accomplish More.* She maintains that "Giving your mind a command to stop thinking is as futile as giving your heart a command to stop beating."

Another resistance to meditation? The idea you must sit in a particular position for it to be effective. What if I told you some of my best meditations were in a recliner chair sitting mostly up, but legs relaxed extended out in front of me? I cannot even sit cross-legged due to the lack of flexion in my knees. It certainly did not exclude me from participating in mediation. I make my rules, as do many others. The avoidance of taking part in meditation all together is of much more concern than the posture you choose.

If you are worried meditation takes years to learn, worry not. Meditation can be learned in a short time. As with anything else, the more you do it, the more you learn what is most effective for you. The notion of perfection is counter-productive.

There is an abundance of techniques and *hacks* for developing a meditation habit. For some fun and simple ideas on starting meditation, see the end of this chapter.

Becoming truly resilient comes with the options various exercises and powerful techniques and practices. Meditation, mindfulness, and breathing are exceptional to integrate into your healing process. I wish I had implemented these paramount tools at the onset of my illness. Regardless of when they came into my life, they were all instrumental in my healing, as well as my ability to maintain my health continuously. The science is robust, the history is lengthy, and the benefits are astounding. There is no justification for not giving it a shot.

Breathing Exercises

Over the years, I have learned about and adopted various breathing techniques from performing them at conferences, workshops, guided meditation practice sessions, or one on one teaching scenarios. You can start by picking one of these and throwing it in at a red light when you're driving. Or insert a session at your desk during the day. Maybe use one as a quick start to your day to get your body set up for success.

Box Breathing:

1. Find an uninterrupted space for at least four minutes.
2. Sit up straight, feet on the floor, hands in your lap. Maintain an aligned posture and be at ease.
3. Close your eyes and dim the lights.
4. Close your mouth and breathe in through your nose. Count to four as you inhale. Hold your breath for four seconds. Allow your belly to move in and out.
5. Open your mouth and exhale for a count of four. Hold the exhale for another count of four.

6. Repeat the exercise for four minutes (or two to three times) to achieve a more relaxed state, to relieve tension, and to settle your nerves.

Alternate Nostril Breathing:

1. In a comfortable position, hold the right thumb over the right nostril and inhale deeply through the left nostril.
2. At the peak of the inhale, close off the left nostril with the ring finger, then exhale through the right nostril.
3. Continue the pattern alternating the inhale.
4. Use for times of focus and energy. This breathing exercise is designed to clear the channels and make you feel more awake.

Progressive Relaxation:

1. Close your eyes.
2. Focus on tensing and relaxing each muscle group for two to three seconds each.
3. Begin at the toes and feet.

4. Work up through the knees, thighs, rear, core, chest, arms, hands, neck, jaw, and eyes.

5. Breathe in and hold on the contraction of the muscle, breathe out on the release.

2x Breathing:

1. Breathe out for double the number of seconds that it takes to breathe in.

2. Breathe in for two counts, exhale for four counts. Repeat three to four times.

3. Breathe in for three counts, exhale for six counts. Repeat two to three times

4. Breathe in for four counts, exhale for eight counts. Repeat two times.

Mindfulness Exercise

For myself, the simple practice of gratitude (see chapter 9) is a mindful exercise. This is my daily commitment to myself, as it not only keeps me shifted to positive aspects of daily living, it also allows me to always see the grace and blessings in my world.

However, various other mindful exercises can be a portal to meditation.

Five Senses Exercise

This is a great one to focus on one main concept – the senses. I experienced this first hand at an Upgrade Labs Conference which focused on Longevity. I also found this formal practice through a positive psychology program [25] and feel it is one of the easier practices to adopt as compared with other mindfulness techniques.

- Notice five things that you can *see*.

  Look around you and bring your attention to five things that you can see. Pick something that you don't normally notice, like a shadow or a small crack in the concrete.

- Notice four things that you can *feel*.

  Bring awareness to four things that you are currently feeling, like the texture of your pants, the feeling of the breeze on your skin, or the smooth surface of a table you are resting your hands on.

- Notice three things you can *hear*.

Take a moment to listen, and note three things that you hear in the background. This can be the chirp of a bird, the hum of the refrigerator, or the faint sounds of traffic from a nearby road.

- Notice two things you can *smell*.

Bring your awareness to smells that you usually filter out, whether they're pleasant or unpleasant. Perhaps the breeze is carrying a whiff of pine trees if you're outside, or the smell of a fast-food restaurant across the street.

- Notice one thing you can *taste*.

Focus on one thing that you can taste right now, at this moment. You can take a sip of a drink, chew a piece of gum, eat something, notice the current taste in your mouth, or even open your mouth to search the air for a taste.

The breathing exercises can also impact a mindfulness activity. Using the breath, in conjunction with other mindful practices, is a fun way to find joy in your training.

Meditation Exercises

"Meditation is much like exercise. The first time you do it, it may be uncomfortable and you may get a little bit sore. One workout for minimal time won't get you in great shape, but working up to a consistent time and frequency will get you in the body of which you dream!"

Like I mentioned at the beginning of the chapter, meditation is becoming mainstream. Pretty soon, if you do not meditate, you won't be one of the cool kids. Maybe not in my lifetime, but mark my words, it has become a "thing." However, everyone who wants to participate needs to find their way into the world of meditation. Some general rules I have learned over my years of developing my practice are:

- There's no room for judgment
- There is no right or wrong way to do it
- You may not feel an amazing impact with every session
- There's no such thing as "clearing your mind" of thoughts

- You get out of it what you put in; essentially, consistency and time are the most powerful contributions you make to your practice
- The idea of perfection is counteractive
- A little bit goes a long way

To start a practice, you simply have to begin. It doesn't matter if it is for a minute at a time. Sometimes using a tool is a helpful way to develop a pattern. There are so many unique ways to practice meditation, but I will focus here on a few that might help get you moving in the right direction. Oodles of resources are available online and you can even purchase some devices that can measure your efforts.

- *Headspace or Calm app*

  Sometimes a simple app can get you started. With our smartphones attached to our hips these days, apps are accessible, brief, and can be used in almost any setting. Both of these have programs and various options that make meditation fun and easy.

- *HRV – Heart Rate Variability*

Compatible with the "Inner Balance" app, the HRV HeartMath Inner Balance Bluetooth sensor or wired sensor is a device that attaches to the earlobe to get a reading on your brainwaves. It uses guided meditations to improve meditation practice. It also measures heart rate variability. It is a brain trainer that helps "shift and replace emotional stress with the emotional balance in coherence."

I invested in a sensor for HRV monitoring and I enjoy it, especially on airplanes and in settings where I can visually observe my heart patterns as thoughts come and go from my mind. It offers a visual breathing rhythm that helps you to tap into your heart cadence so you can learn to influence your body's reactions.

- *The Muse*

This headband is like a Fitbit for your brain. Using EEG technology, the device gives you feedback on your brain's activity during a session of meditation.

The cool thing about the Muse is that you focus on the melody of birds in the background of

246

soundscapes that resemble particular settings: a beach, a city park, a desert, or other locations. When your brain is going in the direction it is supposed to go for optimal meditative response, the birds are more frequent and audible. However, when you get distracted, the birds are non-existent and the noise of the beach waves, thunder or distractions of a busy park chime in and become louder, shifting your focus back to listening for the birds. The Muse also measures your ability to redirect after a distraction. Some people may have the strong re-centering capacity, while others may be better able to be less distracted for longer periods.

After using several weeks of Headspace, the Muse helped me break into my next level of meditation. I first discovered the device at a Bulletproof Labs conference in California. I bought it to help me develop a steadier habit of meditating. I accomplished my goal in the first few months.

- *Meditation Podcasts*

As I have mentioned, I am a sucker for a good podcast. Little did I know that you can pretty much find a podcast on any topic. I don't recall how I found *Meditation Minis* with Chel Hamilton, but I fell hard in love with it shortly after my experience with the *soul journey*. This guided podcast is hosted by a hypnotherapist with a very soothing voice. Her earlier podcasts were filled with creative scenes in which I found myself going to places in my mind I had no idea existed. I had some very powerful meditation sessions using *Meditation Minis.*

Currently, I find *Tune Into You* to be a bit better for independent practice (as opposed to guided sessions). As my practice evolved, I found myself less reliant on guidance and instead of craving some silent time for my mind to do its thing. This podcast allows for both. Each episode is typically around ten minutes, and you can save them and use them over and over. For example, the hostess, Jennifer Davoust, might walk you through a forest and up to a stream of water and ask you to revel in the reflection, choosing someone you love to see looking back at you. You then are asked to imagine looking into a mirror and expressing that same love to yourself as you would to the loved one from the water reflection.

It's amazing how the same scene can create very different experiences in your mind. You can even recall some of the best moments and create your journey from the experiences you found impactful in other mediation sessions. For example, I can now take myself through various scenes of previous guided sessions in my silent sessions.

- *YouTube*

  Similar to the style of a podcast, YouTube offers hundreds of meditations with any theme or style you like. I enjoy these when I would like to go on a long journey or just to change it up now and again.

Remember, there is no wrong way to do this. Pick a time, set up a distinctive place that does not represent an area that you are typically doing other activities that may be stressful, and start. Some days you may have more time than other days, but even just a few minutes can provide substantial gains.

People are using meditation more and more as stress in our society is becoming increasingly problematic, which has a hand in chronic health issues. Just like stress can contribute to the cause of a diagnosis, managing stress through these exercises can help to unravel its impact. Stress is a distinct aspect of POTS and getting the nervous system under control is one of the biggest keys to eliminating symptoms. In the next chapter, I discuss gratitude, which is another way to minimize stress, among other positive benefits.

CHAPTER 9

LITTLE THINGS ARE BIG THINGS – EMBRACING GRATITUDE

"Be grateful for what you have; you'll end up having more. If you concentrate on what you don't have, you will never, ever have enough."

- *Oprah Winfrey*

Gratitude is a magical gift. When you begin to practice it, your life will change.

Gratitude is a substantial step in not only healing but changing your experience along the way. When handed the POTS diagnosis, many are low on hope. They feel like crap. People with POTS get used to feeling like crap. They are focused on all that has gone wrong. They are used to getting no answers and little direction on how to progress through an illness.

But I've found that if they begin to implement gratitude as early as possible in the process, they start to feel better about their situation right away. By the later part of the coaching relationship, they are seeing things through a different set of lenses. Gratitude is an immediate win.

Gratitude quickly changed my view from a cup half empty to a cup half full. Yes, it's the clichéd *look at the bright side* concept. Except it works.

When I had major surgery on a torn hip labrum and detached hamstring, I woke up from surgery only to be instructed I had to wear a tie around my waist that connected to the back of my ankle. This position would keep my leg in a slightly bent position. I called it my hogtie.

I wore this contraption for eight weeks while confined to a walker. I was literally tied up. I lived alone and had two dogs to take care of, one of which had colitis and suffered many accidents. My mom was gone and my sister had her family to take care of. I hired my dog sitter to stay with me for a few days.

Man, it was hard to find gratitude during that time. There were some moments that I am still surprised I was able to work through. However, I practiced every single day. I wrote the following in my journal:

- "I am grateful the universe has slowed me down, so I can learn patience."
- "I am grateful I could walk myself to the bathroom today without knocking anything over."
- "I am grateful I did not spill anything today."
- "I am grateful it took me six minutes to hop to the kitchen, rather than ten."
- "I am grateful Mia did not throw up today."

I did this daily. I created a mindset I could use to get through this period with grace.

There was a reason I was facing the challenge, I knew, and I would look for every opportunity in the experience. I reassured myself repeatedly that I would be bionic after I completed my physical therapy.

At the start, when I imagined two months on a walker, I was completely freaked out and did not think I would survive it. But by taking it one hobble at a time and focusing on the great things I could still do, I got through each day.

Chronic illness, of course, is different from a sports injury. With POTS, it took me a long time to see my condition as a blessing and an opportunity to be grateful. But when I began to look at each day and see promise, I realized how much worse it could be – and each day, I was able to accomplish something with ease became a celebration.

Before my diagnosis, I was so used to feeling lousy that lousy became my normal. Going to work with a slight hangover each day was part of my routine. Now, I know I can expect better. Today, I am grateful POTS changed my lifestyle. Being sick made me a healthier person. It made me mindful and appreciative of my body. It made me aware of how good it feels to feel wonderful. I am also grateful that POTS drove me to change my career. It motivated me to go from selling drugs to helping people get off of them.

Gratitude is a game-changer. One simple mindset shift can change your life. I learned this and so did my clients. The ability to recognize there were still wonderful things in life despite their circumstances kept them from allowing the tough thoughts to hold them down.

Once you begin practicing gratitude, adversity is less exposed. It's not because it does not remain, but because the focus has shifted to something that brings contentment peace, and/or joy.

THE SCIENCE OF GRATITUDE

Gratitude is more than just a mindset shift. Years of research on the topic of gratitude asserts it is the key to psychological and even physical well-being. Look at the evidence:

Gratitude May Be Good for Your Heart

A 1995 study published in the *American Journal of Cardiology* found that people feeling appreciation have improved HRV (heart rate variability), which is an indicator of good heart health. The study was interesting in that it established that anger produces a sympathetic or fight or flight response while gratitude induced a parasympathetic or a more calming effect. [26]

Gratitude May Help You Sleep Better

Studies suggest sleep may be positively impacted by practicing gratitude. In a study of 401 people with forty percent reporting sleep impairment, the more grateful people reported falling asleep more quickly, staying asleep longer, feeling they had better sleep quality, and seeing an improvement in daytime wakefulness. [27]

Gratitude May Boost Your Self-Esteem

According to a 2014 study published in the *Journal of Applied Sport Psychology*, grateful people can appreciate others' accomplishments, reducing social comparison.

Gratitude May Improve Your Mental Health

Studies involving nearly 300 people, mostly college students seeking mental health counseling for issues related to depression and anxiety, revealed that patients who participated in counseling along with gratitude writing had significantly better mental health four weeks and twelve weeks after the exercise. [28]

Gratitude May Increase Your Patience

Northeastern University researchers found that people who were grateful for the everyday little things were more patient and better able to make sensible decisions, compared to those who did not feel gracious on a day to day basis. [29]

Research backs up what I've seen in myself and my clients; practicing an attitude of gratitude is one of the simplest ways to improve your life. But where do you start?

HOW TO PRACTICE GRATITUDE: START BY BREAKING FROM THE NEGATIVE

When I coach clients, often they ask me, "How do I just start thinking positively when I have spent most of my life looking at the negative?" My answer is always "practice." Gratitude isn't instant. You need to pay attention to how much negative chatter may be consuming your brain. If you aren't in tune with the fact that you may be swimming in doubt and self-judgment, you may not recognize the need to shift your focus to something you value, rather than criticizing. Once you are aware of your thoughts, you can begin to shift to alternative ways of looking at a problem or situation.

After achieving awareness, follow up with repeated effort practicing the feeling you *want*, rather than what you don't want. We pay way too much attention to our thoughts and less to our feelings. Ask yourself, "How do I want to *feel?*" Many people feel stress or anger or frustration when they only want peace, calm, or ease. Reminding yourself of what feeling you are seeking will bring about more attention to things that create that feeling in your world.

I had a client who was a self-proclaimed pessimist. She couldn't get out of her way. Everyone around her was an "idiot" and she confessed she hated humanity and people. Her tolerance for daily interactions was very small. When she explained she and her husband were buying a home and it was all a mess and a horrible process, I identified this stressor as a great opportunity to practice gratitude.

We first created examples of finding gratitude for the people with whom she was stuck dealing. In this case, we started with the inspector of the property. She explained how "dumb" he was. In an attempt to reframe, I explained it must be difficult for this person to do well in a job and work in that field if he was lacking education or intellect. I asked her to offer compassion rather than anger towards him, as we never know what is happening in someone's life that leaves them curt with others. She changed her view and decided she was grateful for her intelligence. Compassion can instigate gratitude in most circumstances.

Next, we looked at the owner of the house on which she and her husband were bidding. The owner was driving a hard bargain. My client was angry at what a terrible person she must be. She was able to reexamine the situation and decided she would be grateful for the outcome because if she did not get this house, there was a reason. She realized there were many things about the house she did not truly love, and in the end, she became appreciative of the deal's failure to go through. It became

259

clear to my client that this failure was a blessing in disguise.

Using this one situation to practice daily gratitude over time, my client found herself becoming the "positive one." Her ability to go with the flow was incredibly improved. She told me her husband had always been the level-headed one, but he had swiftly become the worrier and more of the stress now showed up in him. We laughed as I told her she had been stressing enough for both of them before – now it was nice and balanced.

Practicing gratitude in this way is critical. Remember, if you have spent most of your life up until now practicing negative thought patterns (and most of us have without realizing it), this step will require even more awareness and training. But you'll get there.

Now that you've seen how gratitude works in others, it's time to flip the script for yourself. It's not going to be easy. Most people are comfortable with their chaos. When you live with a pattern of consistent negative thinking, the anticipation of catastrophe, and predicting dire outcomes, it would be more *uncomfortable* to feel peace and calm. You may not know what to do with yourself if you had nothing to complain about.

Also, you've invested a lot of time into practicing negativity. Undoing that pattern will take time and effort, in part because you have to fight your brain to do it. Our brains love certainty. We are programmed for survival and certainty ensures survival. Tony Robbins' work with over 3 million people has resulted in his maintaining that humans are driven by six core needs, certainty being the first because it satisfies the need for safety, security, and predictability, and it provides you with the promise you will either evade pain or acquire pleasure.

Remember that repeated thoughts turn into beliefs. We get these thoughts and beliefs from various places: our parents, our observation of others' experiences, societal influences, and our personal experiences. When we believe something so strongly we accept it as fact, our brains will seek out experiences that will reinforce that belief.

For example, a health-related belief might be, "I've tried everything. Every diet, every doctor, every online program, every exercise program has failed me. I am certain nothing is going to work to get my health back

261

on track." If you walk into a coaching or doctor relationship with the predicted outcome that "This will never work. Nothing ever works," the chances of your getting the outcome to support your certainty is great. At the end of the process, you can proudly say you were right. It didn't work. You then reinforce that belief in your lack of health success by repeating that pattern over and over:

You have an off day: "See, it's not working."

You feel good: "It's a fluke, I won't feel good for very long."

You argue for your limitations: "I can't take supplements, I can't exercise, I can't, I can't, I can't..."

The reason we do this is we have all of these stories in our minds that we have developed over years, many of which we concluded after we misinterpreted the facts of a situation and turned them into repeated thoughts, which ultimately became our "limited belief."

If you're still in the headspace of negativity, ask yourself: "How often am I feeding my brain good information, positive affirmations, and self-compliments?" The answer for most of us is rarely, if ever. Most of us would never speak to a friend the way

262

we speak to ourselves. Yet we continue to berate ourselves and our abilities, and then somehow wonder why we're not feeling more optimistic about our potential to get better and feel healthier.

Gratitude is a way to keep yourself coming back to a place of love and compassion for yourself and others. It allows you to focus on the things in your life that are favorable. I always ask my clients "what's great?" or have them make a note of their daily "wins." These are both simple expressions of gratitude. Why not give it a try? After all, negative feelings aren't helping you; no amount of cynical thinking or stress will produce a smoother outcome.

Sometimes the very things that knock us down are the blessings in disguise. Sometimes things aren't always laid out in a cookie-cutter pattern. On the road to better health and wellness, you are going to get lost or be redirected. You'll take the scenic route, get flat tires, and hit speed bumps and traffic jams. There's a bigger plan, and the moment we realize we can surrender the perceived control we think we have, that's when the magic is revealed. Don't give up dreaming; let the process of reaching the dream play out in God's way.

Exercise: Practicing Gratitude

Gratitude changed my life. I practiced gratitude in different ways. You may want to experiment with both morning and evening. The morning allows you to begin your day with an attitude of appreciation. The evening helps to reflect on your day. Try keeping little journals around in the car, by your bedside, in the kitchen, anywhere you may want to make a note. You can also insert gratitude for things in your life that might not have happened yet.

- In the evening, write down at least three things for which you are grateful. Once you get going, you may find, as I always have, that your list will keep going well beyond three things.

- Throughout the day, practice gratitude – especially during times of stress or boredom. I start during peaceful morning walks with my dogs, Poshy and Bucky, but I also practice during the most stressful times in Florida traffic.

- For example, some days I express my awe of nature. I like to say the things I love about the blue sky or the birds chirping out loud. This puts me clearly in the present moment and it allows me to revel in the beauty.

- Other times, I may find myself with my heart pounding because someone just cut me off. The moment I realize I want to curse angrily and possibly add a hand gesture, I instead take a deep breath and recognize that it was a good thing I was paying attention. Or I choose to be grateful I am not in a rush, so that person who is can go ahead of me. I also say to myself, "I do not know the person's circumstances." They may be rushing to the hospital to be by the side of a loved one. I would never know. This reflection gives me a feeling of compassion rather than anger.

- When you find yourself being repetitive or going through the motions of gratitude, take it up a notch. Instead of listing three simple things, list one thing and select five reasons why you're so grateful for this person or experience.

For example, I am grateful for my sister. Why?

  o My sister always looks out for me and includes me in all of her family events.

o My sister has the kindest heart and the most thoughtful gestures.

o My sister makes an effort to make me smile when I am down.

o My sister tells me the truth, even if I don't want to hear it.

o My sister has an amazing sense of humor and I laugh every time we are together.

When you begin looking for the good in all situations, suddenly you find yourself uncomfortable with anything negative. It becomes harder to find things in your life that is *worse* than it is to come up with something that makes you feel blessed.

Gratitude is a game-changer. As we transition into chapter 10, consider where gratitude fits into your new story.

CHAPTER 10

PLANT SOME FLOWERS IN YOUR POTS – CHANGE YOUR STORY

"Our goal is not to ignore the problems of life, but to put ourselves in better mental and emotional states to not only come up with solutions but really meet the challenges and take action."

– Tony Robbins

My orthopedic doctor has reminded me that I have the knees of an eighty-year-old since I was in my twenties. This is another diagnosis I find myself wearing like a badge of honor if I don't pay attention to my inner dialogue.

267

I have lived with stinky knees for most of my adult life. It's my normal. But it is not who I am, it doesn't define me, and even if I am riding out this set of wheels until I am old enough to get a new set, most people aren't aware of this drawback. I work to keep them in shape and I use the mindset tools to divorce my diagnosis.

Separating yourself from your diagnosis may not change the look of an x-ray or the results of a blood test, but neither one of those measurements is reflective of who you are as a person and how you may choose to live your life. For someone with POTS, it is difficult to understand how powerful it can be to keep those things separate in your mind – until you change your story.

This takes effort and practice because you've invested years – perhaps your entire life – into telling that story.

WHERE DO THE STORIES BEGIN?

We are constantly designing both general and elaborate stories about ourselves from the time we are young children. Originally, they may come from outside influence. For example, a parent could be disregarding their child who is trying to get their attention by staring at a cell phone and ignoring him. That child may decide that "I am not important." Or perhaps an unintended criticism coming from a person you respect – perhaps the person even meant to share it to be humorous – could leave you with the general assumption that "I am not good enough." Or it could be not being chosen for a sports team in elementary school might have left you with the belief that "People don't like me" or "I am not athletic."

Most of us are not consciously aware we are telling ourselves these stories. But the sooner we realize we are, the sooner we discover that our stories might be more in control of our decisions than we think. It's incredible when you begin to connect these hypothetical dots that you may discover, as I did when I explored some of my tendencies to avoid certain emotions.

I learned at a very early age that crying made people worry. After experiencing significant loss as a teenager, one being a brother to suicide, I cried frequently. Because of this, my parents worried about me all of the time.

The following year, I experienced the grief of losing my first love to a tragic car accident. My father was extremely uncomfortable with my outpouring of emotion. Seeing me cry uncontrollably on the day of my beloved's service sent my dad into a state of helplessness and fear. At that moment, he warned me that if I didn't stop crying, I could not attend my boyfriend's funeral.

I built my story at that moment: "It's not okay to cry; people will worry about you."

I didn't cry for four years and cried very rarely after that. My dad wasn't trying to be mean or hurt me. He was simply expressing his grief and fear of losing one child. His truth was dictating his expression to me.

However, this one moment when my story about crying was created carried through my life. I went on to spend most of my early career in a male-dominant environment where emotion was not acceptable. Being unemotional was easy for me by then. It was a safe place for me to hold my feelings hostage. In corporate America, you never let them see you sweat, let alone cry.

These days – years after dealing with POTS and rewriting my stories – I cry all of the time. Indeed, at times I provoke emotion so I can make sure to practice *feeling*. If I have that "lump" in my throat and I know I need a minor meltdown, I may listen to a song, visit the cemetery, listen to a saved voice memo, or read an old journal entry. Whatever it takes to keep my new story alive, which is, "I am comfortable experiencing uncomfortable feelings and express them when they come up for me. It is necessary to release emotion."

These stories are everywhere. You have some of your own. How do they relate to POTS? To discover some of the links to your own stories and identify where you may be practicing a learned, but undesirable habit, begin by working through some of the exercises at the end of this chapter.

IDENTIFY YOUR STORY

Conservatively speaking, the average person has between 12,000 and 60,000 thoughts per day, according to a 2005 article published by the National Science Foundation. Many people would argue there are over 80,000 unconscious and conscious thoughts swishing around our minds on a given day. The article's authors maintain that eighty percent of these thoughts are

271

negative and ninety-five percent of them are the same repetitive thoughts as the day prior. [30]

Yikes! We already know the power of our thoughts and how they impact us physiologically for both the positive and negative. Imagine repeating the same negative thoughts day in and day out. Seemingly, this is what humans do.

These are not always conscious thoughts, of course. If you look at your brain as a database or index of our experiences and thoughts, we have a giant directory of beliefs we have created about ourselves. These may come from our parents, the stories we made up to protect ourselves, our observational learnings, and things we are absorbing from others' statements toward us.

Based on this variety of input, how much would you say is stored in your brain as positive, inspiring, affirming beliefs? How often does your brain scroll through and find a language of assurance and uplifting words?

Our stories are constantly unfolding right before our eyes and we are the narrator. Our self-talk becomes a routine just like other aspects of our day. When we consistently reinstate negative stories, we essentially form a habit as regular as brushing our teeth.

If our thoughts are driving how we feel, then those repeated thoughts will determine how we habitually feel.

CHANGING YOUR POTS STORY

There's a disparity between life before diagnosis and life after. The way you describe yourself and your lifestyle may have been one way and now it is another. The story changed.

A diagnosis can be much like a banner or title. Once you identify with something, you begin to form your story around it.

You believe you used to have freedom, more choices, fewer limitations. Now you consider life distinctively different than it used to be. And it is different. But *you* are the same person at your core. It's very important where you go in your mind during these moments. You can become aware of how you now differentiate the *before and after*. As Norman Vincent

Peale reminds us, "Change your thoughts and you change your world."

Experiences are staples in the formation of our stories. Experience is an event such as being left in a relationship. This experience may leave you feeling a sense of abandonment that crosses over to other areas of your life. These events become integrated with our sense of self. If you can begin to recognize the experiences you have during this new chapter of your life, you may probably be able to develop a story that better serves you for a healthy pattern and healthy behavior now and in the future.

Another example of recognizing the potential for an event to be disruptive was when my Mom passed away. I already held intense fears of love resulting in a tragic loss as it had with my first boyfriend that had been taken so young. I knew if I did not seek help from a therapist and pay attention to this story I was leaning toward, I would live afraid of loving deeply and I did not want that for myself.

Homaira Kabir explains this well: "Identity is nothing but an evolving story that finds coherence with the past, present and future. Find the flexibility in your

274

story that allows you to adapt to changing circumstances, and you'll be able to stand up as authentically "you" through the ups and downs of life."

Every one of my clients holds stories that both protect them and prove to be harmful to living the life they wish to live. I explore how they were able to make these shifts in their beliefs to develop language and patterns of belief that helped them to "grow through are they were going through." Changing your story can be powerful as evidenced by various client experiences, as well as my experience. Where do you begin?

You can change your story by developing awareness. Becoming aware of the stories you tell and the poor self-talk you use is a great starting point. Before you can change these automatic thoughts, you need to see them and recognize them. Sometimes, it's easiest to start by looking around you rather than within you. Noticing this kind of behavior in others will help you to see it in yourself.

Have you ever been around someone who is constantly criticizing themselves? I used to work with a girl who described herself as overweight. Even after she lost the weight, she would consistently make fun of herself any shot she had by way of telling jokes about her size or shaming herself with humor. The problem was, her criticism of her weight wasn't funny nor was it accurate. Her self-image had not shifted; she still identified as being the heavyset woman.

When I witness people shame themselves like this, it makes me physically uncomfortable. If it is a friend, I will point the negative self-talk out so they can be aware of the words they just used as a weapon against their character.

We have to speak to ourselves as we would speak to a friend. Heck, most of us wouldn't allow friends like the ones that live in our heads to be a part of our lives. Yet we allow ourselves to do significant damage daily without even acknowledging we are doing it.

Simple awareness is crucial. When you catch yourself going down the rabbit hole of critique, use the various tools below to break this habit.

Tool #1: Create a Vision

Earlier in this book, we talked about one of the first steps you must take to overcome POTS: imagining the life you want. To move forward, you have to envision a desirable outcome. Create a vision of a life that will serve you and support your desire for healthy and happy existence.

You must be able to see yourself feeling well. You must *believe* in the prospect of enjoying life again. We tend to get stuck in the belief that this is it; this is our new reality. That mentality has to shift. Your diagnosis is not your destiny!

Visualization is one way to make this shift. Interrupting yourself is also valuable. When you hear yourself talking unnecessarily about your diagnosis in everyday conversation, remind yourself of your new story. You may do this by creating an affirmation like, "I am healthy and strong." Alternatively, you may have a mantra that helps get you through tough moments and puts you back on track. I often use "onward" when I feel like I am overthinking something that is done that I cannot take back.

Continually practicing these corrections begins to shift your focus on what you desire rather than on your symptoms. Remember: this is a *practice*. It takes time and needs to be done in combination with the other critical steps.

You also need to *imagine* the new story. Really feel it. Where do you see yourself? Get specific. Develop the details and all of the nitty-gritty of how you feel in this new version of you.

Adopting this way of thinking may be hard at first. Some people are not as in tune with their bodies as others and they don't realize the control they have over their mindset.

When I started thinking like this, I was so aware of my body, I could almost predict how I would feel moment to moment. I could not control what would provoke my symptoms, but I knew I could control my reaction and more importantly, my attitude. I could let it stop me or I could let it drive me harder.

There's a fine line between truly separating yourself from POTS and believing you are in control. Believing you are in control reminds you of your ability to rule your perception and the attention to which you give to your diagnosis. Separating yourself without accountability for your role can still leave you floundering.

278

When you change your story, you are choosing to focus on the things in your life that bring you confidence and pleasure. You avoid the stories that are holding you back because they are full of grief, disappointment, fear, and certainty of a poor outcome.

You also de-emphasize the diagnostic label and reclaim your true identity. We do this for others, who've been ill; why not for ourselves? Not once do I think of my mom as the woman who had cancer. Nor do I remember my dad as the guy with diabetes. Have you ever lost a loved one and only recalled their diagnosis rather than all of the beautiful memories of who they truly are and what they meant to you? Their cause of death has nothing to do with how they lived their lives. They are the amazing, courageous humans who have a much bigger identity than the title of a disease.

So are you.

Tool #2: Flip the Script

What comes next after awareness and creating a vision? Changing your relationship with POTS starts with changing your language.

After I decided to stop calling POTS *mine*, I intentionally chose to go about life as if nothing was wrong whatsoever. Similar to the situation of my arthritic knees and the Celebrex, I coached myself through the mental discomfort.

I knew my body. I knew the discomfort of symptoms. But I also knew that the symptoms pass. So, why give them more energy than they deserve?

When I wanted to use the word "POTS," or when I experienced the symptoms, I simply acknowledged the condition and moved forward, rather than harping on the fact that they showed up again. I used to stir in all that I could have done differently to avoid the symptoms. I would attempt to make adjustments to *fix* them through medication or some type of tool. This was no longer my instinct.

I did this by repeating to myself:

- "I am not POTS" "I acknowledge the presence of my body talking, but I choose to proceed without pause."
- "I chose to focus on feelings of health and joy."
- "I chose to change my story."

I am not saying it is *easy* to say these things and believe them. But what choice do you have? Look at it this way: by speaking the illness into existence and thinking about the symptoms, everything you notice becomes exaggerated. The headache may become more profound. The fatigue turns on the brain fog. This noticing does not improve how you feel. It makes it worse. Now your attention is creating more energy around the "problem."

Instead, changing the dialogue with yourself can be like magic. It can instantly shift your attention to a place that brings you restored faith.

Simply shift the focus to how you *wish* to feel. Don't tell yourself what not to feel. ("I want this pain to go away.") If you tell yourself not to focus on a thing, what happens? You focus on it more! Instead, shift your focus on what you *desire* to feel, not on what you don't desire. Directing yourself to focus on something alluring you want ("My head is clear and I can finish reading this book") is much more effective than instructing yourself to stop feeling something you don't want.

Whether the diagnosis exists or doesn't exist for you, life proceeds the same way. Harping on its actuality, acknowledging it, engaging with it, and allowing yourself to dwell on all the things that came with it doesn't do any good. Your life continues whether you do all that or not.

I learned after Mom passed that life simply must go on, even when you don't want it to. Even when you just need the universe to freeze for a few days. People go about life; the world still turns. You can stay still and become paralyzed by your pain or fear. Or you can put one foot in front of the other and take one day at a time, one moment at a time. It's okay to realize life will not always be rainbows and butterflies, but you can create a land of beauty in your mind to get you through the tougher moments. As Friedrich Nietzsche said, "He who has a why to live for can bear almost any how."

Exercise: 3 Practices to Change Your Story

Practice #1: Thought Replacement Exercise

Remember the mental Rolodex, that database of thoughts that your brain has access to when it is searching for certainty? Your brain can only search for and find thoughts that live within that database. But what if your database is 100 percent limited beliefs, sad stories, or thoughts you want to outgrow? Wouldn't you want to give your brain something confident onto which it can grab ahold? You can – by adding new thoughts to your database.

I use a technique with my clients introduced to me by the work of Lisa Nichols. It's called *Exposing the Lies*.[31] I primarily look at the health and wellness category, but this exercise can be done with various aspects of life: health and wellness, finance and business, relationships (romantic and familial), and spirituality and faith. It's an exercise that can provide significant breakthroughs if you stick with it. Here's how you do it:

1. Take out paper, a pencil, and a red pen. Plan for as many pieces of paper that it takes.

2. When you begin to have negative talk, what are some of the things you tell yourself? Write them down. Without editing. This is the "lie," the limited belief.

3. Skip four lines in between each thought (or lie) you are telling yourself. The thoughts that move

283

you to a place of fear, sadness, or frustration or personal disappointment about a person or situation.

4. Repeat. Write as many thoughts as you need to. Keep dumping each lie onto the page. Try not to deal with it at that moment. Just get it out. Expose the lies. The more you fill-up, the better you are. You may feel yucky during this time. It is not easy.

5. One by one, in the space underneath, in red ink, write down what you know to be the truth, even if you can't believe the thought yet. The red is going to be the new data for your brain to retrieve when you attempt to repeat the lie.

6. Read the lie, followed by the truth, at least three times over every day for seven days. Forming a thought replacement between the pencil statement and the red ink will create a new connection in your brain. Continue this practice for 30 days.

7. Last, erase the lies you wrote in pencil. The sentences in red that remain are the script for your new self- talk.

Your brain will begin to toggle between the lie and the truth. Eventually, the brain will auto-correct these thoughts, creating patterns of positivity built by the replacement thoughts. When the chatter returns, your new neurolinguistics pattern will emerge, and the red will stand out more than the pencil. Now you have something to invalidate the lie.

To practice this exercise as it relates to your diagnosis, an example of the "lies" and "truth" may be:

Limited Belief: I can't exercise because I have no energy.

Truth: Energy begets energy. When I move, my body grooves. Movement generates energy.

Limited Belief: I am going to struggle for the rest of my life.

Truth: POTS does not define me. My life is better because of POTS because I am aware of my body and the need to fuel myself with healthy foods and positive thoughts. I take care of myself.

Limited Belief: I am not a good parent because I am sick.

Truth: I lead by example. Putting my energy into my healing makes me better so I can take care of the people that I love. When I am well, I have more to give to others. I cannot pour from an empty cup.

Practice #2: Improve Awareness by Prefacing Negative Affirmations with "up until Now…"

I learned this technique from a remarkable therapist with whom I worked after my dad died. In our initial calls, when I spoke of myself in ways that I wished to change, she would remind me that "up until now":

- I have always been closed with my emotions.
- I always do _____ .
- I was rigid in my thinking.
- I feel lousy if I don't do _____ .

You get the picture. Using this phrase was an excellent way for me to catch myself defining my "ways," which were based on my story at the time. By creating this prologue, I was required to stop and reframe my statement. Putting "up until now" before these statements profoundly and changed the meaning and added an immediate assumption this was something I *used* to do in the past.

Practice #3: Imagine Your Best Day Ever

Write down every emotion you feel on that day. Include actions you take, the detailed scenery, how you feel in response to the energy, the weather, the sunshine, the rain, whatever that day looks like for you. What will you eat? How will you move? Simply expressing this through writing will etch it into your thoughts, followed by memory, and eventually belief. Keep this description handy and read it often.

Think about expanding on this. What does your best life look like in five years? In ten? Even twenty? Record yourself reading your best day ever, along with your future in five, ten, and twenty years.

I adopted this practice after working with another therapist who helped me to get out of my way. While we practiced so many techniques and strategic ways to retrain my brain, this simple recording process was the most powerful. In the past, I had written about my future repeatedly, but putting this vision in my voice and reading it "as if" it was already in progress made a bigger impact.

I still have a recording of me and my projected future. I love listening to it. I explicitly describe how it feels to walk pain-free in high heels. I exercise without breathlessness. I can eat freely some of the foods I could not consider during POTS. With precision, I talk about how much joy, comfort, security, abundance, calm, certainty, and love I feel in my day. I designed scenes of where I am going, who is by my side, and how the ideal life will feel when I stay the course and continue to improve myself. It is on the voice memos of my phone so I can reach for it as often as I like.

It's time to get tired of the stories that are dragging you down. It's time to create new ones.

Through practice, repetition and time, you will find these new stories become your new belief system. Consistency will create the changes you are seeking. Remember, it takes practice to identify with the new story you have realized to be your truth. After all, we have spent years relying on the stories that have kept us cemented in place. We are comfortable there.

The opportunity to practice these exercises in an ongoing fashion will allow you to witness yourself creating the stories as you go along. This process will allow you to identify which stories will be helpful and which ones will hold you back from your best you. When you change your POTS story, your experience of life changes. The next chapter will help you decide how you will put all that you have learned into action!

CHAPTER 11

PICK YOUR PAIN

"Adversity is the first path to truth."

- *Lord Byron*

Now that you have been introduced to the critical steps that carried me from POTS back to freedom in my health, what will it take for someone to establish the discipline and habits to implement these tools consistently?

I have read countless books and attended dozens of seminars only to return home to my normal routine and set aside all that I had learned. Even the most incredible and simple habits were left on the table because I did not spend the time and effort on an online course or following up on the vigorous notes I had written down with each speaker. I did not dedicate myself to the processes that were so abundantly available to me.

Walking the walk is always more effective with a coach. I may have developed the POTS skills through the process of elimination and self-experimentation, but it took many years. Today, I lean on my therapists, coaches, trainers, and I work one on one with the best in their trade.

Take exercise, for instance. I like having a trainer to tell me what to do. Sometimes, I need to be out of my mind and just do what I am told to do. It gives me a break from over-intellectualizing everything! I also like to go to group classes so that I can absorb the energy in the room and know that the people around me are facing the same sweaty struggle as I am. Pilates is a class where my friends all meet up. It holds me accountable because if I don't show up, I can expect several phone calls asking where I was. When I am in a funk, I am called out. When it is raining, I refuse to lose money by not making it to class. If I feel tired, I know going through the motions will draw out my energy.

However, the story I have always told myself is that I *can't* work out at home. I stand by that story. Except I would change it to say, "I choose to not work out at home because I enjoy the connection I have with my fitness community." I have a bike at home, a Pilates machine, a full gym set up, including a Bosu ball, kettlebells, weights, yoga equipment...you name it. It doesn't change the fact that when I have a coach to hold my hand, the accountability of friends, and a trainer to tell me what to do so I don't try to do too many things at once – I am successful in my fitness. It's great to have the workout room for back up, but let's face it, I don't use it.

WHEN LIFE HAPPENS

When each of my parents passed away, the horrible grief presented as a set-back. I used exercise and my team of people to get my heart back into life. I am forever grateful to these people. They kept me from falling back into a POTS hole.

I have clients that could completely fall off track with their health practices. Life is going to *happen at you* all of the time. Nothing is ever pure highs or constant lows. It ebbs and flows. There will always be something that will scream "set back!" This is just a fact of life. Every single day you will be faced with stressors and challenges, some are conceivable and others are unimaginable. How will you stay true to your POTS journey? These are the stressful times when POTS wants to rear its ugly head and try to take you back behind that speed bump once again.

Staying on track with completing the steps outlined in this book takes discipline and consistency. It takes time to adopt the habits and it takes encouragement. POTS does not make it easy by any means. Just when you think you are in control, something happens that reminds you to keep up your guard. You are going to have days when you don't feel like being a cheerleader for yourself. On some occasions, you will feel like accepting defeat. When you have the steps to fall back on, you will always know you can pick yourself back up from whatever fall you may take.

But what if you don't follow the steps? This book then becomes another dust magnet on your shelf. You'll tell yourself you tried everything. You will practice an exercise or two, a time or two and resign that this is not going to work for *you* because your case is *different.* The principles in this book have been applied and tested across illnesses that varied from Type 1 Diabetes, Crohn's disease, chronic pain syndrome and several cases of cancer. Every case is different, but the concepts of healing all came back to these consistent actions. You will find cases that may be much worse than yours and others that may be heaps easier than what you are dealing with in a diagnosis of POTS. Not to mention, POTS is often not a solo diagnosis. It goes hand and hand with many other chronic illnesses that hold a gigantic battle of their own. Addressing POTS is only one piece of the puzzle, but these practices apply to a variety of conditions.

You will want to quit. You will want to make excuses. You will feel stuck at times. You will stop at times. Yet on other days, you will feel like you can climb mountains.

WORK WITH A COACH

The option of working with me, the author, the POTS Expert (amongst other things) is available to you. Taking each step in stride with a coach, consultant, encourager, and tribe member can make everything more doable. I am there to believe in you when you lose faith in your body and health. It is the sense of ease you get and feel when you know you have someone whom you can ask questions about your personal case. Working with me will give you the confidence of knowing how to get back to living your dreams without taking too many wrong turns and wasting too much time and energy that is so much better used in settings that serve a joyful purpose. The steps are not just concepts, they are weekly action-items and are focused on measurable outcomes. The final chapter will help you decide if you are ready to truly get out from under POTS and get back your true identity!

CHAPTER 12

DIVORCE YOUR DIAGNOSIS

"A person is so much more than the name of a
diagnosis on a chart."

- *Sharon Draper*

Have you ever received some advice you just knew was bad? When I worked in a corporate job, one of my co-workers was very arrogant and full of ego. Customers either loved him or hated him. I inherited some of his accounts, and when I asked him about one of them, he replied, "If it ain't broke, don't fix it."

I thought, "Hmm, I don't know about that."

In sales, I felt I needed to be proactive. I liked to make sure I did things that benefited customers before they had to come and ask me because a competitor was trying to beat me to the service. I liked being one step ahead of their needs, rather than being reactive when things fell apart. That was simply paying attention.

I took the piece of advice my co-worker gave me and went out of my way to ignore it. I did just the opposite.

The same thing applies to health. I was broken, and I fixed it. But to stay in one piece, I continue to proactively stay on top of my health *before* I may be faced with another physical challenge. If you function from the old saying, "If it ain't broke, don't fix it," you're stuck in the gap between being healthy and being diseased. Remember John F. Kennedy's words? "The time to fix the roof is when the sun is shining."

Most people wait until the day they're diagnosed or when they suddenly experience symptoms. They hear the whispers of their body but then they wait until it screams at them before they take action.

We take care of our cars, upgrade our iPhones, and invest in our homes often better than we commit to our bodies and minds. Every day people wake up and think, "I'm going to start that diet tomorrow," "I'll try to

298

meditate this week," or, "I'll watch less television next week."

The problem with this mindset is tomorrow never comes. They continually make choices that do not support their health goals. They do things to their bodies they know are not optimal. They put in the bad and take out good instead of the other way around. That puts a giant gap between themselves and good health until they are in a full-blown diagnosis or disease state.

What happens on that bridge from healthy to sick is what matters. You don't just start on one side and hop to the other. All the things you do in between keep you on the left side of the continuum. It's much harder to reverse once you have crossed over the halfway point to disease than it is to be proactive about staying on the left side of the progression through life.

This book explains to you how to *know better*; now you can *do better*. By faithfully practicing the daily habits in spite of POTS, you'll find the possibilities are endless. You can create goals that expand beyond just having your health. You can go back to experiencing life. You have more power and control over your mind and body than you could have imagined. Your cells are listening to your thoughts. Your thoughts are driving your beliefs.

I wrote this book because had I had access to a resource that provided me these tools when I was first diagnosed or even at my all-time lowest with POTS, I would have saved myself years of suffering beyond what was necessary to take on the challenge of the diagnosis. I would have saved myself years of medications damaging my body further when I only thought I was helping it along. Even just knowing how I could have supplemented to offset the negative sides of the drugs would have kept me in a more stable place and allowed for quicker healing. If I had found functional medicine earlier in my journey, I would have had the tests that revealed the puzzle pieces that pointed to my root cause(s) of POTS.

At the end of the book, my wish for you is that you find hope in healing. You realize POTS is not who you are and it no longer has to be your identity.

Throughout the chapters, you have learned how I was able to solve the POTS puzzle for myself and others. I understand the challenges with POTS; I know how to get the symptoms under control and often free them up completely. You have learned how to take responsibility for your role in your health to find your answers instead of fully relying on doctors and outside sources and why it is important. You have learned how to keep your records and follow trends.

You have learned that to feel well with POTS is not just dependent on the fuel you put into your body, but also prioritizing sleep, managing stress, and moving your body. Supplements have a big place in today's society of nutrient depletion and supporting the malnutrition caused by pharmaceutical drugs. You have resources and general principles that promote wellness to support your initiative to feel better.

You now know the significance of the people in your life playing a positive, uplifting and supportive role will change the course of your experience with POTS. Being selective with your *tribe* gives you the help you need to power on. There are multiple ways to find connections to the people most need to attract into your life and it is not always in person that provided the influence.

You are now empowered to be proactive, educated, and embrace all of the information needed to

301

support your personal growth and healing. You can walk into a doctor with more information on the latest research than he can offer. You understand where to find credible resources and don't waste time, money or energy relying solely on other people directing your path.

You have found harmony in the times when you may need to fake it until you make it, while also honoring your body, respecting the reality of POTS, and moving through the emotional aspects of healing. This understanding of the need for both brings you to a place of *true resilience*.

With an intentional gratitude practice in your routine, you can now shift the focus from the reality of the illness to the things that in life that are wonderful. You cannot be depressed and grateful at the same time.

You are now aware of the stories that are not serving you and by simply identifying them, you can unravel those stories to create more powerful truths that support healing. You have exercises that help you to continually work through this throughout life's challenges and celebrations. Knowing the triggers that drive your behavior puts you in the driver's seat.

I was reminded of the impact of these practices just recently when faced with a traumatic, sad, and stressful situation. I was cruising along quite comfortable in my life when my relationship came to a screeching halt after almost two years. This happened just three days before my birthday. I was flooded with feelings of confusion and sadness. Just the following week, my sweetest boxer dog, Mia, passed away suddenly. I was devastated and now grieving two substantial losses. My first instinct was to acknowledge gratitude. I recognized the fact that Mia died suddenly and did not suffer was a blessing. I was grateful she passed on her own without my having to make a horrible decision like I was forced to do with my past two boxer dogs. This brought me peace.

In my mind and body's search for understanding, I still found myself feeling overwhelmingly depressed. My default mood and state had become one of happiness. I lived a happy life in spite of things around me so it was very uncomfortable to feel this deep sadness. I allowed, I cried, I honored my need to lay low, while also recognized my need for connection and close friendships. I immediately knew I had to take it all up a notch. I needed more meditation time, more time with my tribe, and extensive gratitude practice. I had to pay exceptional attention to my nutrition and exercise as the tears were depleting my hydration and the stress was messing with my hunger hormones. I begin creating my story around the break-up. Would it be a story of abandonment or one of a beautiful stepping stone with great memories and lessons I could take on to the next chapter of my life? I had to choose. It was my decision how long I would remain in that place of desperate loneliness.

I loved how powerful the tools had worked for me in my life and especially in these moments. It wasn't POTS haunting me this time. But the stress of life can always knock you off course, prompting your body to go into fight or flight (POTS favorite place to live).

My wish for you is to believe and find hope that you can conquer POTS symptoms. I hope that you are inspired by the success I have not only felt in my personal experience but also have witnessed in patients with POTS. There is a quality of life to be had. You can now disengage from POTS and not let it rule your life.

You have steps to take that can be used to improve on many areas of your life.

Take these insights, apply them, and watch your life change!

ACKNOWLEDGMENTS

First, I'd like to thank my sister, Kristin, for always encouraging me when I called her in a panic trying to figure out if I was investing in the right things. Thank you for always saying "go for it" and for never letting me turn back. Thank you for loving me so much.

To my friends, my never-ending supporters, my mentors, my soul sisters who never stopped encouraging me; each one of you played a very specific role in my completion of this book. Thank you for listening to the struggles, always asking how it was going, and for your sincere interest in the answer.

Special thank you to Patti, my proof reader who took the time to not only read, but dog-ear, highlight and provide the feedback I needed to have the courage to publish.

Thank you to my clients who work so hard to change their minds and body. You are the warriors who navigate daily through their health struggles, but never give up: the bold souls who don't take no for an answer.

Each one of you has a unique superpower that the world is ready to receive.

Thank you to my editor, Kristen Havens, with whom I worked before going in a different direction and focusing solely on POTS. She was critical in teaching me about writing.

Thank you to my parents for teaching me integrity, strength, character, love and that I can do anything on which I set my mind. You gave me wings. I love you dearly.

ABOUT THE AUTHOR

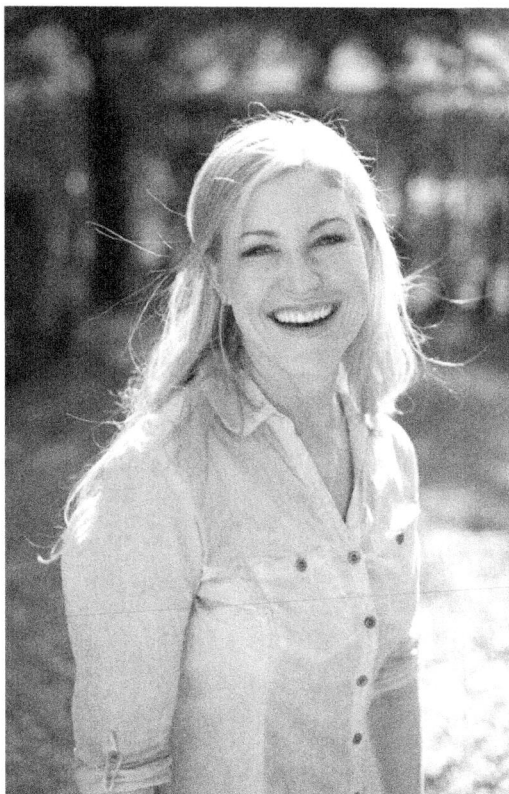

Leslie Harrington is a transformational health coach and diagnosis strategist who helps people to get their life back after being diagnosed with chronic illness. She empowers them to be their own advocates, work effectively with their practitioners, and make lifestyle, dietary, and other self-management changes necessary to have a quality life in spite of a diagnosis.

Leslie has a master's degree in mental health therapy and uses the connection between mind and body to understand the dynamics of the human spirit and the ability to live with vitality and get better with age. Her primary motivation for making an impact on the world is to create an organization in her mom's memory. The *Love Like Laurice* Project will be dedicated to raising money for various organizations supporting children.

Leslie is a native Floridian. After losing her brother to suicide, she took an active interest in mental health. She completed her degree in psychology at FSU and her graduate degree in mental health therapy at Nova Southeastern University.

She became certified as a transformational health coach through the Institute for Transformational Nutrition, which includes psychological and spiritual aspects of wellness, addressing transformation above and beyond nutrition. She also earned her certification as a functional diagnostic nutrition practitioner through Functional Diagnostic Nutrition, which offers functional lab training and data-driven protocols to help people on

310

a deeper level using labs to identify healing opportunities.

Her successful and ongoing eighteen-year career in the pharmaceutical industry gives her a unique view of the world of medications and how using food as medicine can be more powerful and safe than most commercial prescription drugs.

She works one-on-one with clients and also does group coaching through her independent business from her hometown of Davie, Florida. She worked as a health coach at Vida Integrative Medicine in Sunrise, FL. Leslie has developed a step-by-step process to address all aspects of wellness including and beyond exercise and nutrition. Her primary client base is those diagnosed with postural orthostatic tachycardia syndrome (POTS) as she was able to overcome the symptoms of POTS after her diagnosis over ten years ago.

It wasn't until her diagnosis that she disconnected from the conventional medical system and was consistently disappointed with the overly prescribed medications and lack of interest in finding what caused the breakdown in her body. After witnessing her mom's tragic passing from cancer and her dad's erosion from heart disease and diabetes, she became incredibly passionate about health.

Leslie loves her dogs, Posh and Bucky, (and sweet Mia who was by her side through it all before her passing in 2019) Pilates, and fresh flowers. She looks back on her diagnosis and realizes it happened for her, not to her. It enabled her to not only get healthy herself but to help others realize their diagnosis is not their identity. She believes no diagnosis has to define a person's destiny.

Website:
http://leslieharrington.net/
Email:
admin@leslieharrington.net
Facebook:
https://www.facebook.com/leslie.harrington21
Instagram:
https://www.instagram.com/laharrington72

THANK YOU

Thank you so much for reading *POTS Is Ruining My Life: The Ultimate Guide to Finding Freedom from the Symptoms of Postural Orthostatic Tachycardia Syndrome.* If you've made it this far, I know one of two things about you: first, you're more ready than ever to experience life after POTS. Second, maybe you also start at the end of the book before diving in (hey, me too!).

I would love to learn more about your journey and experience with managing symptoms of POTS. Please keep in touch (I'm most active Facebook and Instagram), and share your wins (tag me and use #divorceyourdiagnosis).

314

REFERENCES

1. Dysautonomia International. (2019). *Postural Orthostatic Tachycardia Syndrome.* Retrieved from https://www.dysautonomiainternational.org/page.php?ID=30

2. Dr. Valentin Fuster (Commentary) 2019, March 2019. JACC [Audio Podcast] American College of Cardiology, *Postural Orthostatic Tachycardia Syndrome.* Retrieved from https://player.fm/series/jacc-podcast/postural-orthostatic-tachycardia-syndrome

3. Lawrence, Guy (Host). 180 Nutrition – Health Sessions [Audio Podcast] The ABC of Functional Medicine – Chris Kresser Expert Interview. Retrieved from https://180nutrition.com.au/180-tv/chris-kresser-interview/

4. MarketResearch.com. (2017, December 20). *U.S. Weight Loss Market Worth $66 Billion.* Retrieved from https://www.prnewswire.com/news-releases/us-weight-loss-market-worth-66-billion-300573968.html

5. Department of Pharmacology, University of Michigan Medical School. Neuropsychopharmacology. (2016, December). *Eating 'Junk-Food' Produces Rapid and Long Lasting Increases in NAc CP-AMPA Receptors: Implications for Enhanced Cue-Induced Motivation*

315

and Food Addicition. Retrieved from
https://www.ncbi.nlm.nih.gov/pubmed/27383008

6. ExtoxNet FAQs. *Metals in Drinking Water.*
   Retrieved from
   http://extoxnet.orst.edu/faqs/safedrink/metals.htm

7. NIH (National Institute of Environmental Health
   Sciences). *Endocrine Disruptors.* (2019). Retrieved
   from
   https://www.niehs.nih.gov/health/topics/agents/end
   ocrine/index.cfm

8. Domonoske, Camila. NPR LRN Miami/South
   Florida (2016, September 13) *50 Years Ago, Sugar
   Industry Quietly Paid Scientists To Point Blame At
   Fat.* Retrieved from
   https://www.npr.org/sections/thetwo-
   way/2019/09/13/493739074/50-years-ago-sugar-
   industry-quietly-paid-scientists-to-point-blame-at-
   fat

9. Trauth, Erin. (2014) One Green Planet. *If Big Food
   Owns Most of the Organic Industry, Who Can You
   Buy From?* Retrieved from
   https://www.onegreenplanet.org/vegan-food/big-
   food-owns-organic-industry/

10. WebMD. (2017, December 10). *The Effects of
    Stress on Your Body.* Retrieved from

https://www.webmd.com/balance/stress-management/effects-of-stress-on-your-body

11. Taheri, Shahrad, Lin, Ling, Mignot, Emmanuel. (2004, December 1) PLoS Medicine. *Short Sleep Deprivation is Associated with Reduced Leptin, Elevated Ghrelin, and Increased Body Mass Index.* Retrieved from https://www.ncbi.nlm.nih.gov/pmc/articles/PMC53 5701/

12. Friedman, Noah, Salter, Lamar. (2017, December 29) Independent. *A Sleep Expert Explains What Happens to Your Body and Brain If You Don't Get Enough Sleep.* Retrieved from https://www.independent.co.uk/news/health/sleep-what-happens-not-enough-stay-up-late-brain-body-science-health-a8133161.html

13. Breus, Michael J, PhD. (2017, November 30). Sleep Newzzz. *Hot Nights Can Disrupt Your Sleep.* Retrieved from https://www.psychologytoday.com/us/blog/sleep-newzzz/201711/hot-nights-can-disrupt-your-sleep

14. Harvard Health Publishing. *Say "good night" to neck pain.* Retrieved from https://www.health.harvard.edu/pain/say-good-night-to-neck-pain

15. Buckeley, Kelly, PhD. (2014, December 14). *Why Sleep Deprivation is Torture.* Retrieved from https://www.psychologytoday.com/us/blog/dreamin

g-in-the-digital-age/201412/why-sleep-deprivation-is-torture

16. Mohd, Razali Salleh. (2008, October). Malaysian Journal of Medical Science. *Life Event, Stress and Illness*. Retrieved from https://www.ncbi.nlm.nih.gov/pmc/articles/PMC33 41916/

17. Clark, Corey M. Rochester Institute of Technology. *Relations Between Social Support and Physical Health*. Retrieved from http://www.personalityresearch.org/papers/clark.ht ml

18. Cockerham, William, PhD, Hamby, Bryant, MA, and Oates, Gabriela PhD. (2017, January) American Journal of Preventative Medicine. *The Social Determinants of Chronic Disease*. Retrieved from https://www.ncbi.nlm.nih.gov/pmc/articles/PMC53 28595/

19. Brown, MJ, Thacker, LR, Cohen, SA.(2013, June 11). Department of Family Medicine and Population Health, Virginia Commonwealth University School of Medicine. *Association Between Adverse Childhood Experiences and Diagnosis of Cancer*. Retrieved from https://www.ncbi.nlm.nih.gov/pubmed/23776494

20. Centers For Disease Control and Prevention. *About the CDC-Kaiser ACE Study*. Retrieved from https://www.cdc.gov/violenceprevention/childabuse andneglect/acestudy/about.html

21. Bolte Taylor, Dr. Jill. *My Stroke of Insight – A Brain Scientist's Personal Journey.* Penguin Books, 2009.

22. Bergland, Christopher. (2017, May 16). Diaphragmatic Breathing Exercises and Your Vagus Nerve. Retrieved from https://www.psychologytoday.com/us/blog/the-athletes-way/201705/diaphragmatic-breathing-exercises-and-your-vagus-nerve

23. Center for Anxiety and Traumatic Stress Disorders, Massachusetts General Hospital. (2013, August). *Randomized Controlled Trial of Mindfulness Meditation for Generalized Anxiety Disorder: Effects on Anxiety and Stress Reactivity.* Retrieved from https://www.ncbi.nlm.nih.gov/pubmed/23541163

24. National Center for Complementary and Integrative Health. *Meditation: In Depth.* Retrieved from https://nccih.nih.gov/health/meditation/overview.htm

25. Ackerman, Courtney E. MSc. (2019, November 21). *22 Mindfulness Exercises, Techniques, & Activities for Adults.* Retrieved from https://positivepsychologyprogram.com/mindfulnes s-exercises-techniques-activities/

26. American Journal of Cardiology, vol 76, 14, (page 1089-1093). (1995, November 15). *The Effects of Emotions on Short-Term Power Spectrum Analysis of Heart Rate Variability.* Retrieved from http://www.laskow.net/uploads/5/7/6/4/57643809/th e_effets_of_emotions.pdf

27. Wood, Alex M., Joseph, Stephen, Lloyd, Joanna, Atkins, Samuel. (2009) Journal of Psychosomatic Research 66. *Gratitude Influences Sleep Through the Mechanism of Pre-Sleep Cognitions.* Retrieved from https://greatergood.berkeley.edu/images/application _uploads/Wood-GratitudeSleep.pdf

28. Wong, Y. Joel, Owen, Jesse, Gabana, Nicole T., Brown, Joshua W., McInnis, Sydney, Toth, Paul, & Gilman, Lynn. (2016, May 3). Journal of Psychotherapy Research. *Does Gratitude Writing Improve the Mental Health of Psychotherapy Clients? Evidence From a Randomized Controlled Trial.* Retrieved from https://www.tandfonline.com/doi/abs/10.1080/1050

3307.2016.1169332?scroll=top&needAccess=true&
journalCode=tpsr20

29. Dickens, Leah, DeSteno, David. (2016). APA Psyc
NET. *The Grateful Are Patient: Heightened Daily
Gratitude is Associated With Attenuated Temporal
Discounting.* Retrieved from
https://psycnet.apa.org/record/2016-15319-001

30. Verma, Prakhar. (2018, May 17). *A Practical Guide
for Positive Thinking (Works Instantly!)* Retrieved
from https://medium.com/swlh/how-to-stop-
negative-thoughts-in-180-seconds-without-
meditating-4ef29cda09d1

31. Nichols, Lisa. *No Matter What! 9 Steps to Living
The Life You Love.* Grand Central Life & Style,
2011.

Printed in Great Britain
by Amazon

70887298R00190